CIVIL WAR NURSE NARRATIVES

AF765887

from September 1862, ...
in the hospitals in and ...
kept a journal of ...
ons of which (that journal) appea...
the journal was kept ...
d not for publication.
to at night when so we...
d mental) anxiety and ...
not unfrequently fall ...
often sat upon a box ...
d held my book on ...
d now this journal, co...
e lap of the public, a...
who have earnestly re...
s White may be ent...

Civil War Nurse Narratives, 1863–1870

DANEEN WARDROP

UNIVERSITY OF IOWA PRESS | IOWA CITY

University of Iowa Press, Iowa City 52242
Copyright © 2015 by the University of Iowa Press
www.uiowapress.org
Printed in the United States of America

Design by April Leidig

No part of this book may be reproduced or used in any form or by any means without permission in writing from the publisher. All reasonable steps have been taken to contact copyright holders of material used in this book. The publisher would be pleased to make suitable arrangements with any whom it has not been possible to reach.

The University of Iowa Press is a member of Green Press Initiative and is committed to preserving natural resources.

Printed on acid-free paper

Library of Congress Cataloging-in-Publication Data
Wardrop, Daneen, 1952–
Civil War nurse narratives, 1863–1870 / Daneen Wardrop.
pages cm
Includes bibliographical references and index.
ISBN 978-1-60938-367-1 (pbk)
ISBN 978-1-60938-368-8 (ebk)
1. United States—History—Civil War, 1861–1865—Medical care. 2. United States—History—Civil War, 1861–1865—Personal narratives. 3. United States—History—Civil War, 1861–1865—Women. 4. Nurses—United States—History—19th century. I. Title.
E621.W25 2015
973.7'750922—dc23 2015005562

for Dad

CONTENTS

ACKNOWLEDGMENTS

I am grateful to the following people who offered invaluable assistance on the project of *Nurse Narratives*: Elisabeth Chretien, Editor, University of Iowa Press; Michelle Ganz, Archivist, Special Collections Librarian, Lincoln Memorial University Archives, Abraham Lincoln Library and Museum; Sharon Carlson, Director, Archives and Regional History Collections, Western Michigan University; Donna Eschenbrenner, Archivist, The History Center in Tompkins County; Lisa Murphy, Archivist, Kalamazoo College Library; Rachel Ingold, Curator, History of Medicine Collections, Rubenstein Rare Book and Manuscript Library, Duke University; Julie Hayward, Manager, Resource Sharing, Western Michigan University; Susan Steuer, Head, Special Collections and Rare Book Room, Western Michigan University; and Jeffrey R. McGranahan, Collections Manager, Historical Society of Montgomery County. I am especially grateful to Western Michigan University for a sabbatical leave that allowed me time to work on this book.

I have charge of the diet—assist each meal in dealing it out. I have covered crutches, ripped up arm slings, washed and made them over, gone to commissary with order from doctor for material for pads for wounded or amputated limbs, and manufactured the same. I petition, and thus commence the transfer or furlough of one or the pay of another. I write letters for my patients, read or sing for them, visit or play checkers with them ... been allowed to make some cake as a treat. ... In short, have tried to make my ward look as Miss B. expressed it, "as if there was a woman in it."
—Elvira Powers (128)[1]

These notes were jotted down as the incidents occurred; they are a simple statement of facts simply stated.
—Julia Dunlap (xiii)

INTRODUCTION

Given the historically unprecedented situation of female nurses working in hospitals, the women who decided to chronicle their experiences during the Civil War took on the considerable task of describing and justifying their labor. Women nurses entered an 1860s workplace both strange and familiar: strange, in that they had traveled far from a hometown, often for the first time, to enter an unknown city or camp to tend to soldiers, and familiar, in that they gave care to the sick as they did to family members at home. Publishing narratives in the clutch of war and soon after, they recorded interactions with patients, wardmasters, stewards, cooks, laundry workers, officers, privates, freedpeople, Native American soldiers, other female nurses, male nurses, Northerners, Southerners, patients' family members, doctors, surgeons in charge, and townspeople. During the years 1863–1870, Union women nurses wrote and published twelve single-authored narratives that chronicled their experiences in relief work. These narratives detailed in an informal, readable rhetoric the everyday demands they encountered during the turbulent mid-century years when American culture underwent social changes in gender, race, ethnicity, and class.

Civil War Nurse Narratives examines the writing strategies that seven of these twelve narrators used to recount their work experiences: Louisa May Alcott's 1863 *Hospital Sketches*, Georgeanna Woolsey's 1863 *Three Weeks at Gettysburg*, Julia Dunlap's 1864 *Notes of Hospital Life*, Elvira Powers's 1866 *Hospital Pencillings*, Anna Morris Holstein's 1867 *Three Years in Field Hospitals of the Army of the Potomac*, Sophronia Bucklin's 1869 *In Hospital and Camp*, and Julia Wheelock's 1870 *The Boys in White*. The narratives, to a greater or lesser extent, foreground the personal development of the narrators,[2] each of whom represents different working conditions. Louisa May Alcott and Julia Dunlap each served only in one hospital, Alcott in the cramped Union Hotel Hospital in Washington, DC, and Dunlap in the Episcopal Hospital of Philadelphia, Pennsylvania, her city of residence. Georgeanna Woolsey worked in the field at Gettysburg, and Elvira Powers, from Massachusetts, traversed the country to serve as far south as Tennessee and as far west as Indiana.[3] Anna Morris Holstein labored less often in hospitals than in camps—some of those bordering directly on the front—and Sophronia Bucklin was stationed in several locations, at one point positioned so near the front she could hear "the screams of shells and the whiz of bullets" (285). Julia Wheelock worked mostly in the greater Washington, DC, area of Virginia and Maryland, visiting various facilities because of her position with a state relief association.

These were just seven of thousands of women who tended to soldier-patients. More than 20,000 women served during the Civil War, historian Jane Schultz asserts[4]—an estimate that certainly falls short, given that it includes only Union nurses who were paid and on the record; Schultz

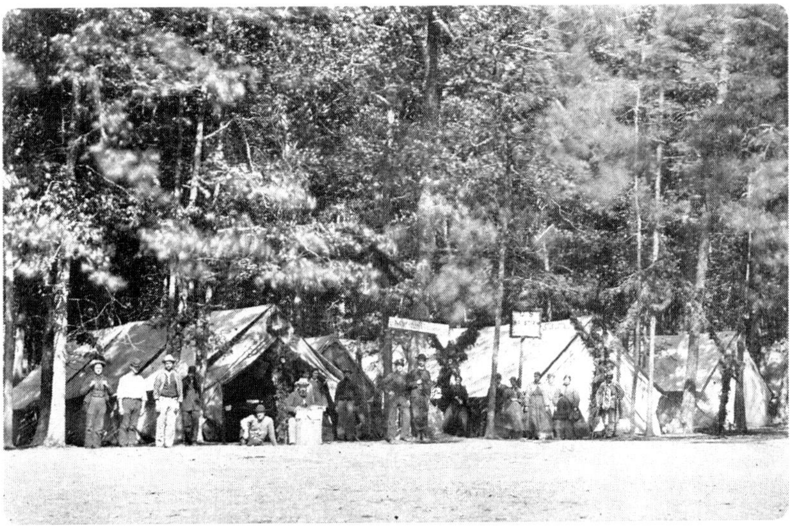

Christian Commission at Gettysburg General Hospital, 1863

Courtesy of the Library of Congress

offers the caveat that the total was "*undoubtedly much larger*" (Schultz 20).[5] Jane Stuart Woolsey, Superintendent of Nurses at Fairfax Seminary Hospital, identified the large number and heterogeneity of Civil War female nurses to include both "paid and unpaid" workers, relatives of patients, friends who "remained without any clear commission duties," those assigned by General Superintendent of Nurses Dorothea Dix, and those employed by state agencies and aid society women (Woolsey 41). In other words, the influx of female nurses can be attributed to their being hired by Superintendent Dix starting in 1861 and their working under the auspices of the two largest relief organizations—the United States Sanitary Commission (USSC) and the United States Christian Commission (USCC)—as well as for many state relief organizations. In addition, nurses included sisters from the Roman Catholic church, freedpeople who were taken into Northern camps, and family members or friends who arrived to care for their loved ones and stayed on to serve patients. Female nurses came from many different backgrounds, divergent in terms of class and race, and took on the labor for widely varied reasons.

Prior to the Civil War, women cared for family members at home, but rarely in medical institutions. Nurses outside the home typically were male convalescents or former patients who continued service in a civilian hospital because they were indigent.[6] As for military institutions, few existed, because in antebellum years the military for the most part ran small dispensaries on forts. The staggering number of battle casualties at the outbreak of the Civil War necessitated an improvisation of facilities for medical care, so that the wounded were attended in makeshift stations such as churches, hotels, warehouses, and even for a while in the United States Patent Office (Brockett and Vaughn 113). After the battle of the First Bull Run, the United States government suddenly and urgently needed nurses to care for the wounded, and American women followed Florence Nightingale's inspirational example[7] of nursing soldiers during the Crimean War of 1853–1856.[8] Women entered Civil War duty by traveling to hospitals hastily set up, sometimes in disarray, with unclear or shifting chains of command. At hospital camps they confronted similar difficulties, along with the additional dangers of being at times in proximity to battles. In 1862 the Federal government began to construct institutions that would provide large-scale medical care and by the end of the war operated 204 hospitals that cared for more than one million Union soldiers (Wagner 627–28). Nursing duties, far from systematized, especially in the first years, included the varied work of overseeing medicines and diets, bathing soldiers, writing letters, reading to soldiers, cooking, laundering, and cleaning; in some hospitals and camps, women nurses assisted at surgeries and dressed wounds.

This study concentrates exclusively on Union nurse narratives, because the dynamic for Confederate nurses proved markedly different, partly because Southern women published fewer narratives (one-third as many), given that the publishing industry in the South dwindled under the Confederacy.[9] Moreover, since many battles occurred on their home turf, Southern nurses faced a different social construct than their Northern counterparts, who usually traveled to the site of a new work location. As Nina Silber observes, Southern women were often "closer to the chaos of the battlefield, frequently subjected to the constraints of Union occupation, and often shaped by the trauma of defeat" (*Battle* 7).

Union and Confederate nurses experienced divergent physical, social, and psychological circumstances, a variation that demands the respect of contrasting analytical treatment for Confederate nurses.

In the seven brief years from 1863 to 1870, nurse narratives came to define what this project determines to be a subset of war literature that continued—after jumping the decade of the 1870s—into the 1880s and early twentieth century.[10] During the hiatus of the 1870s, the American populace recovered, with those who survived wounds and disease undergoing rehabilitation, communities rebuilding their businesses and institutions, and broken family structures regrouping.[11] The nurse narratives that reappeared in the 1880s were more reminiscent, sometimes polemical, and compromised by nostalgia: "Increasingly conciliatory in tone as memory of the war receded, narratives after 1880 seldom mentioned sectional enmity and were less critical of the military administration of hospitals" (Schultz 7). For the most part these later narratives demonstrated a measured acceptance of loss and embraced commemoration. Hoisington states, for instance, that the Woolsey family's correspondence several decades after the war reflected this softened tone: "The perspective of thirty years tempered many harsh judgments" (Hoisington xix). Women writing after the war took a more measured perspective, as did even Alcott when she revised her 1863 *Hospital Sketches* in an 1869 version that took a less harsh view, for instance, of Rebel soldiers.

This project, then, concentrates on the first wave of the narratives, published in the decade of the 1860s, to showcase the potent narrative strategies nurses used to achieve a fully dimensional chronicling of their experience during the major conflagration of the United States. The central inquiry of *Civil War Nurse Narratives* focuses on how nurse narrative strategies were informed by rhetorical tactics conceived through antebellum United States social movements, and how those tactics were adapted for the purpose of exerting influence with readers. Nineteenth-century rhetoric proved instrumental to nurse memoirists developing their own narrative voices, enabling them to construct a powerful bond with their audience. I advance *Civil War Nurse Narratives* as the first book-length study to examine texts published during this brief and crucial moment of American history, texts that not only represent the nascent hospital labor of women but stand as literary memoirs with their own discursive merits.

Of the seven narratives, some have received vigorous scholarly attention and some less so. The works of four of the seven authors—Julia Dunlap, Anna Morris Holstein, Elvira Powers, and Julia Wheelock—have seen relatively little treatment and no comprehensive scholarly essays. For instance, Dunlap's *Notes of Hospital Life*, which describes her work in the Hospital of the Protestant Episcopal Church in Philadelphia, has drawn few comments, other than that she was the anonymous narrator of the work, until 2010, when her name was verified.[12] Dunlap's memoir is examined here in the light of Philadelphia church documents and other sources to ascertain how the church was involved in defining her hospital position to clarify the nature of her benevolent work, and to further authenticate her identity. Anna Holstein, the semi-anonymous author of *Three Years in Field Hospitals of the Army of the Potomac*, was published by Lippincott, the same press that published Dunlap 's work, and both women were acquainted with Philadelphia Bishop Potter. Powers's *Hospital Pencillings*, a book of verve and perception, which has likewise seen thin scholarly traffic, is examined in this project through Episcopalian documents and through her correspondence with Frank Moore, editor of the 1866 *Women of the War*. Julia Wheelock's *The Boys in White* describes her service as an agent for the Michigan Relief Association in Washington, DC. Her work is analyzed in detail through a cross-reading of her narrative with her diaries, manuscript, and scrapbook to demonstrate how she framed her memoir.

Of the three more familiar narratives, Louisa May Alcott's *Hospital Sketches* is available in several editions and has been widely studied along with the extensive biographical materials available to scholars. To understand her narrative as the combination of humor and pathos that renders it a kind of literary tour de force and a touchstone of cultural and historical importance, it is tracked through its early reception, through contemporaneous reviews, and reader responses. Georgeanna Woolsey's *Three Weeks at Gettysburg* has warranted attention primarily as it spoke to her sisters' and her contributions to the field of modern nursing and as it satisfied human interest in the prestigious and influential New York

Woolsey family. This project supplements historians' understanding of the Sanitary Commission's promotion of Woolsey's narrative to increase further reader reception and attract further donations. Sophronia Bucklin's *In Hospital and Camp*, which has been examined to date in several critical works, is addressed through further scrutiny of the manuscript version of her narrative and of her letters and other personal papers, which clarify her resistance to bureaucratic inefficiency and graft and her affinity with the rank-and-file.

BEFORE SPEAKING IN MORE DETAIL of the rhetorical and narrative strategies used by these memoirists, the political and social arenas the nurses inhabited during the Civil War must be contextualized. *Civil War Nurse Narratives* argues for the intrinsic importance of three major nineteenth-century cultural concerns that were paramount to the United States as a whole and, of course, to the narratives. The nurse memoirs propose refinements and enrich our understanding of these three mid-century concerns: women's rights, interracial interactions, and the development of a national character.

The first concern—the tracking of women's rights—arises from the fact that nurse memoirs addressed the "woman question" by developing resourceful articulations of women's labor in their newfound jobs as caretakers of soldier-patients. Women's involvement in activism necessarily changed during the war, when less organizational activity was devoted to the cause of female advancement. Concerning the mid-century women's rights movement, Catherine Clinton asserts that, "the impetus gained by women's apprenticeship in the antislavery, temperance, and purity movements was no match for the Civil War" (*Other* 80–81).[13] Similarly, Judith Ann Giesberg argues that there was a shortage of organizational activity for women's rights during the mid-century years (the key activity occurring during 1820–30), with the important exception of the United States Sanitary Commission, a group formed specifically to give relief to Union soldiers. Despite its male leadership, the USSC formed the "missing link" in women's organizing, for women were prominent in the organization as "the initiators, the main financial supporters and a significant part of the workforce"; they also "set the groundwork for the sweeping reform efforts and the emergence of mass women's politics that characterized the rest of the nineteenth and most of the twentieth century" (Giesberg, *Sisterhood* xi, 12).

I acknowledge Giesberg's assessment that relief organizations such as the USSC were a critical link to women's postwar activism but also assert the importance of individual initiative as a contributing factor to women's rights, precisely through the act of work and the corollary act of writing about it. Women recording their involvement in all aspects of the war, from community organizing to hospital nursing, chronicled it in newspapers, magazines, and books; they articulated the crucial presence of female contributions in supporting the soldiers and the war effort in general. While the women's rights movement advanced through the organizational activity of relief associations, it also progressed through individual initiative stoked by the conviction that a consolidation of rights was manifest in labor and in the written word. The nurse narrator inaugurated a rhetoric of such labor, and her readers were changed by her modeling of female fortitude.

Historians of reading underscore the process of imagination involved in the active consumption of narrative whereby reader character becomes altered. Alice Fahs, for instance, argues that reading was essential to the formation of personality: "War became not just an obsessive, all-consuming subject but also a mode of perception and way of life that disrupted and reorganized authors' and readers' conceptions of identity, nationhood, and even time itself" (18). Memoirs activated audience imaginations when readers compared themselves with women nurses experiencing personal and national quandaries brought on by firsthand involvement in war-related work. The power to envision new scenarios was instrumental in developing political acumen, in that "women's journeys to public identities" depended on "the ways in which reading stirred imaginations and fostered female ambition" (Sicherman, *Well-Read* 1).[14] The imagination's capacity to absorb new perspectives from literary images "was related to the prewar insistence upon the power of moral suasion," a power also "emphatically political—meaning that it participated in the power relations in society" (Sizer 5). With the expansion of literacy and print culture, the number of women readers increased, as did the number of women writers, many of whom chose to write for a gendered audience eager for material.

The nurse narrator felt personal commitment to a patriotism that depended on both male and female input and demonstrated such commitment to the enterprise of hospital service. Nineteenth-century proponents of women's rights set forth resolutions in gatherings such as the 1848 Seneca Falls Convention, but found in the decade or so following that they needed a praxis to correspond to those resolutions. The woman in the hospital workplace developed that praxis. This investigation of nurse narratives published during the span of only several years provides a historical focus between the prewar and postwar years of women's organizing—a slice of time for assessing a gendered testimony of experience in which the nurse narrator deployed rhetorical maneuvers that served to validate female labor and agency.[15]

Nurse narrators not only articulated but lived an ideology of "woman's rights." Among the many liberties proclaimed at Seneca Falls were the right to vote, hold political office, and enjoy equality in marriage, none of which were pursued with organizational vigor during the war. Also proclaimed, however, were "equal rights in the universities, in the trades and professions" (Stanton, Anthony, Gage 73), and the right to pursue meaningful labor was provided in the Civil War, despite the fact, of course, that virtually no jobs for women provided equal working conditions, let alone pay. In previous decades, American working-class women had begun to labor at the Lowell, Massachusetts, textile mills and at other mills under increasingly controversial workplace circumstances, later entering into strikes for better conditions, but in the 1860s most women of all classes and races provided labor, whether at home, in benevolent societies, or nearer the front, for the war effort. Women nurses framed these gendered concerns in their narratives, buoyed by the principles of justice, arguing if not immediately for themselves, then vigorously for their patients, and so by proxy for themselves. Rather than formulating a broad declaration of suffrage, nurses recounted day-to-day difficulties and successes, assessing gender roles as they promoted efficient care for soldiers. Their actions spoke loudly and effectively because they chronicled their labor to an audience crucially invested in the war cause, secondarily because their service formed a kind of proving ground for "woman's rights."

The second cultural concern examined in *Civil War Nurse Narratives* deals with interracial interactions during the years 1863–70. This period, characterized by upheaval in such interactions, was bookended by the Emancipation Proclamation in 1863 and the Fifteenth Amendment in 1870. The Emancipation Proclamation, which held that all enslaved persons "are, and henceforward shall be free" (Beschloss 90), and the Fifteenth Amendment, which guaranteed the right to vote regardless of "race, color, or previous condition of servitude" (Beschloss 109), mark two legal changes that, if not mattering often enough in practice, mattered at least symbolically. These documents heralded legal milestones, though in reality most former bondspeople were still denied freedom, their rights rebuffed through poll taxes, literacy tests, psychological degradation, and acts of physical brutality.

Many white nurse narrators were raised in households where antislavery politics occupied the forefront of family and community discussions. Alcott, for instance, made no bones about being a "red-hot Abolitionist," and Georgeanna Woolsey promoted emancipation in passionate terms, having grown up in a family that "listened to lectures by noted abolitionists such as Wendell Phillips and Dr. George Cheever" (Hoisington xvi). A Woolsey sister reported that she and her siblings "cut our political teeth on the *New-York Tribune*, and were in the right frame of mind to keep step with the steady march to the inevitable through the Kansas perplexities, the John Brown raid and the election of Mr. Lincoln, to the firing of the first gun by the rebels upon the national flag at Fort Sumter" (quoted Dannett 31). Indeed, many women predicated the validity of their Civil War service on the fight against bondage, returning to that conviction when they needed moral uplift. As Lyde Cullen Sizer points out, women abolitionist writers believed fervently that "a war for any purpose other than social justice would not be worth fighting" (102). Indeed, women as a rule felt more comfortable speaking out for slaves than for white women, and organizing to liberate slaves typically took precedence over working to liberate women. Frederick Douglass addressed this discrepancy when he spoke to the women at the Seneca Falls Convention, claiming "many of you who have at last made the discovery that the negroes have some rights as well as other members of the human family, have yet to be convinced that women are entitled to any" (*Selected* 102).

Prompting Northern white women to reexamine the scope of their abolitionist convictions, the Emancipation Proclamation adjusted the direction of political activities from legal concerns to social concerns, from the attempt to end slavery to the attempt to improve the social status of freedpeople. The change required nurse narrators to reassess their approaches to politics because the proclamation, almost overnight, signaled the need to fight the war for justice on different terms—not against slavery as a legal institution, but against racial inequality as an inimical way of life.

Living in hospital communities, white nurses entered into unaccustomed encounters, experiencing social disjunctions that arose from their conception of African Americans as both emblems of and persons associated with abolition; as Quarles and Franklin state, "in the Civil War, the Negro was both a symbol and a participant" (131). White people who had militated for slavery's termination were well-accustomed to thinking of themselves as co-participants in the slave's struggle for freedom but unaccustomed to thinking of themselves as engaged in the fight for equality. In daily hospital life, white nurses often worked side-by-side with black workers and cared for black soldiers; as part of a diverse population of laborers thrown together in the military hospital at the epicenter of shifts in the American politics of race, their antislavery views remained intact, but their own unexamined or skewed conceptions of racial privilege were challenged. Sizer asserts that "white middle-class women" aided their "wronged sisters, both African American and white working class," to "give themselves power and legitimacy," using a "rhetoric of unity [that] was not democratic, despite its claim to a kind of democracy" (11). White women needed to reformulate their attitudes as the country changed and were often unaware that they alternated between fervent political commitment and personal blind spots.

In the twentieth century, Toni Morrison exposed such assumption of white privilege with the phrase, "whiteness and the literary imagination," the subtitle of her vital work, *Playing in the Dark*. Morrison asserts that the history of the United States is founded on the history of race interactions and that public discourse exists in all the "nation's mightiest struggles," precisely with "reference to the situation of its black population" (65). Her recasting of the study of American literature as necessarily the study of racial experience has important implications for this project, in which a large burden of interpretation lies in reading race dynamics and evaluating nineteenth-century American literature to include the "situation of its black population" as it became mobilized in the consciousness of the writer: "I am interested in what prompts and makes possible this process of entering what one is estranged from—and in what disables the foray, for purposes of fiction, into corners of the consciousness held off and away from the reach of the writer's imagination" (4). The nurse memoir can improve an understanding of race dynamics, given that the narrator demonstrates the process of racial estrangement described by Morrison, and approaches, if briefly, inexactly, inconsistently, such new corners of the consciousness in her everyday hospital interactions.[16]

I also draw from analyses of race such as Ruth Frankenberg's *White Women, Race Matters*, which affirms that "race neutrality" is a myth, because "white people are 'raced,' just as men are 'gendered'" (1). White nurses in the Civil War grappled, if incipiently, with their racial identity, at times exhibiting a dawning or intermittent awareness that their actions proceeded not from neutrality but from unexamined perceptions concerning race. Like Frankenberg, Elizabeth Ammons exposes the presumption of white neutrality, calling it "white escape-hatching," an attitude that precludes introspection and thereby any resulting response or action; she, too, calls for literature to examine the harmful "practice of perpetuating white privilege" that is continued exactly by "exempting whiteness from serious race analysis" (ix). As Ammons states, white people have "remained safe from self-confrontation" in a "no-analysis" zone (Najmi x). As evidenced in these early Civil War nurse narratives, some white nurses began to question their assumptions and behaviors of presumed privilege, and such questioning warrants serious study.

As nurses came partly to realize their complicity in racial disparity, they uncovered views not as socially responsible as they had previously assumed. Homi Bhabha sets the critical bar for analysis of racial interactions when he writes that, "the subversive move is to reveal within the very integuments of 'whiteness' the agonistic elements that make it the unsettled, disturbed form of authority that it is" (White 21). While the 1860s racism that emerged in the inadequate rhetoric of unity unfortunately was the norm, dissatisfaction with that norm occasionally did surface; some white nurses tracked their limitations, which allowed them to make at least tentative movements toward progressive changes.

The third cultural concern addressed by *Civil War Nurse Narratives* is the development of a national character through narrative—a development tied in this study to the history of the book and American reading. The power of narrative to build national character informs this project either overtly or tacitly throughout, whereby the nurse memoirist used cultural forces to create a specifically female United States persona. Jonathan Arac, for example, asserts that the prevailing narrative during American literary history from 1830 to 1860 was the "national narrative" (3).[17] Such narratives of developing national character continued to emerge throughout the Civil War, eliciting a democratizing genre that provided the expressive scope for individual Americans to tell their tales and the publishing industry to encourage a print culture dependent on them. The publishing industry grew radically in the early part of the century: during "a time of relatively stable prices, the value of books produced rose from $2.5 million in 1820 to over $16 million in 1865" (Machor 18–19). This explosion in production inspired many women authors who saw an increased opportunity to make the shift from writing privately, in diaries and letters, to writing publicly. Accordingly, they expanded their power to influence a readership, and though not citizens legally, they became citizens in practice as they weighed in on civic duty. With this growth came the opportunity to recount stories that advanced the national narrative by including greater access to the female point of view.

Authors of many narrative genres found avenues for influence, character studies becoming the coin of the realm in the publishing business: "Nineteenth-century citizens grew to develop a "biographical imagination," fed by "a proclivity to see individual lives as stories" (Casper 14).[18] American publishing had always included memoirs, from the seventeenth, eighteenth, and nineteenth centuries, when individuals possessed of singular tales recorded their experiences. The earlier accounts were penned both by people of social rank whose stories garnered interest because of their powerful positions and by those of little social rank who related tales focused on individual progress through a set of trials. By the beginning of the nineteenth century, circumstances became more favorable for the latter, as "Americans were coming to see that the lives of both the noble and the ignoble not only had literary merit but also, as lived experience, had the shape of stories" (Fabian 2). The narrators of less privileged lives, for example, were converts, captives, bondspeople, common soldiers, indigents, and prisoners, all of whom trained the American eye to a more affective accounting precisely because their authenticity depended on less than patrician origins. Such narratives dilated on personal accounts that sometimes mirrored the values of individuals or small communities, thus augmenting the sense of a many-faceted national character.

Stories related by those with diminished social power often could hold fascination for a general readership because they offered actions that were laudable in unconventional ways and modeled the more complex behaviors that accompanied the difficult ethical options available to those without social clout. Such texts invited readers to respond on an emotional level, as they chronicled unusual incidents and sometimes extraordinary adventures of interest to a wide reading population. Reading these accounts became a popular pursuit during the nineteenth century, one intrinsic to the American spirit and significant to the development of a new mass culture: "At this period, reading took on a new significance and a new urgency in the formation of individual, communal, and national identity to the point where it became a recurrent topic—directly or by implication—in the vehicles of an emerging mass culture of public discourse" (Machor 3). The project of the narrative depended on the development of both American character and American culture, and each magnified the other.

Enter the nurse narrative: likewise directed toward a general readership and built on tales of adventure, this new discourse employed the power and popularity of the personal account to dramatize the viability of the project of women performing invaluable labor for the country. Asserting that women nurses embodied a fresh perspective on American identity, this narrative chronicled small personal interactions that were part of a large era and amplified female experience as part of the national mission. The nurse memoirist wrote to readers who welcomed individual experience as a valid part of the historical record. A surfeit of histories existed during the war, and for the most part they were written not by scholars but by "popular historians" who spoke to large numbers of readers who found in them "not dispassionate narration and analysis of the causes of war . . . but an 'enthralling story' that often affirmed the Union's sense of moral righteousness" (Roberts 147). The conditions of the nurse's work sparked the formation of the memoir's distinctive woman narrator who seldom lost sight of the nation's social causes, her place in them, and the popular reception of both. Nineteenth-century readers held the conviction that there was not just one story of any given incident but "a culture-wide sense that all war stories were valuable—whether at the home front or battlefront" (Fahs 14). The cultural cachet of the individual tale at this point in history became a kind of a staple of authenticity in the nineteenth-century perception of historical events.

While the publication industry in general declined, the publication of war literature, specifically, flourished, especially in the form of biographies, histories, war poetry, songs, cartoons, and other works focusing on the conflict: "The New York-based trade journal of the book-publishing industry, for instance, commented in 1862 that though the country was 'engaged in a civil strife which one would suppose would have the effect of draining and absorbing' or at least 'restricting the domestic market,' the opposite was the case" (Fahs 10). Nurse narrators published their books during this singular business climate of the 1860s, when a small window of opportunity opened up for books about the war. War literature, indeed, provided the grist for the industry during the 1860s, thriving not only on battle histories and biographies of officers and politicians but also on accounts of representative people such as the common soldier, whose contributions to an accumulating conception of the national character were essential; memoirs by women nurses offered the female counterpart of the soldiers' accounts. Narratives such as

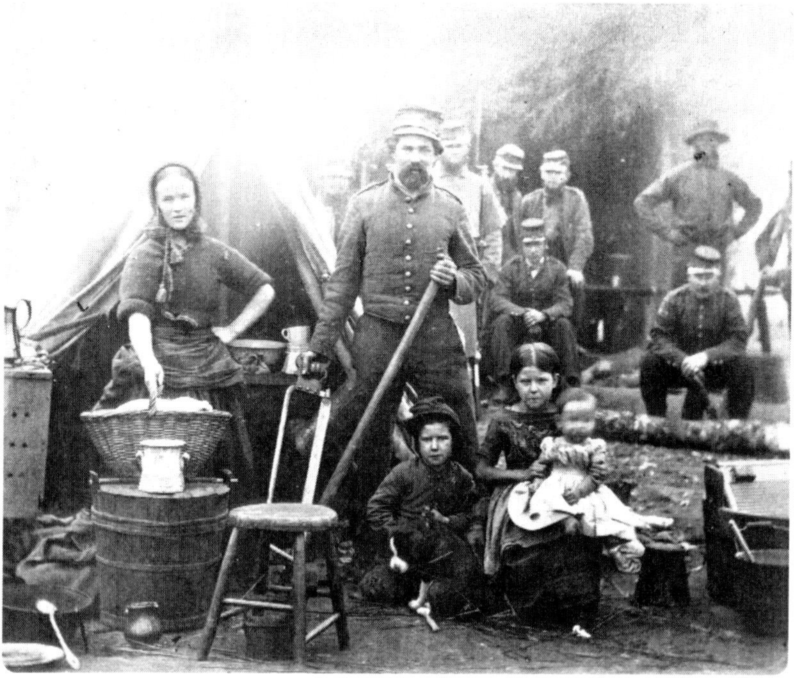

Camp of the 31st Pennsylvania Infantry near Washington, DC
Courtesy of the Library of Congress

Louisa May Alcott's 1863 *Hospital Sketches*, for example, poised perfectly on this upswing in the production of national narratives.

The nurse memoirist related rich and sometimes transformative experiences concerning the cultural constructions of gender and race, situating herself, albeit in understated ways, as a type of the American writing a national narrative. Books by female nurses filled the need to portray women coming to terms with the American project of liberty and cast the narrator in a first-person voice as a major actor in the war drama of freedom. All of the nurse memoirs were patriotic, and all demonstrated at least some aspect of acting in the spirit of women's rights, if still within the parameters of subordinating or integrating that spirit to the comprehensive needs of the nation. All developed a character in the person of the narrator, specifically female, specifically shaped by the exigencies of war.

The importance of studying the nurse narrative as a subgenre of Civil War literature inheres in its ability to contribute to our understanding of the above three cultural concerns of women' rights, interracial interactions, and the development of a national character. As a complex cultural production, the nurse narrative presented the war hospital as a microcosm of the country and a crucible of cultural upheaval. In an undertaking the American woman had not claimed on such a broad scale before, the nurse narrator declared new social and political avenues for women, and in the process initiated a distinct genus of United States literature. Historian Adam Goodheart argues that the Civil War was not composed of battles with "sides" that were "mechanically obeying a set of sociological and ideological rules" (16), but rather of individuals' actions. That verity is embraced in this project, as each American writer who owned a singular and changing set of politics, ethics, fears, and convictions legitimized the individual's contribution to making history, and as each nurse narrator crafted the figure of the female character who actualized her contribution to the national workplace in part by repositioning the gendered citizenry.

THE OVERARCHING CONCERN of *Civil War Nurse Narratives* is the use of narrative strategies and the rhetoric those strategies draw on, especially as crystalized by the three cultural concerns described above. These concerns are shown in high relief when viewed through a history of the nineteenth-century rhetoric that shaped and inscribed the movements, permitting women the means to articulate, resist, and register their conceptions of national issues. Rhetoric being inextricably linked to cultural capital, women's social gains accrued with their ability to assert themselves through increasingly effective discourse. As Nan Johnson writes, "The history of rhetoric necessarily means that the complicated relationship between rhetorical practices and the inscription of cultural power must be addressed" (*Gender* 1). Social power attends rhetoric, and rhetoric attends the question of who shapes and joins the national conversation and how they assert change.

An escalating scholarship in the last quarter-century or so has aimed at retrieving and defining a history of women's rhetoric—a rhetoric that identifies tactics of discourse as it remediates the "gaps and silences and erasures" attending that history (Andrea Lunsford 3). Though relatively few women in the antebellum period were trained academic rhetoricians, there existed no shortage of women who employed skillful, often informal, rhetoric to reach citizens directly and who addressed with acuity the social issues affecting the American populace. Women produced a body of speeches and writings about various nineteenth-century social movements that testified not only to the verve of women's voices, but to the canny language choices that represented the female self as agent of change. In other words, at the same time that women spoke from their own newly mantled resources, they often accrued new cultural power to speak for women's rights. In the history of rhetoric, women's more diverse tools of articulation have been excluded from recognition, as Molly Wertheimer states in perceiving that rhetoric has been "too narrowly conceived for most of its history and that feminism can provide important kinds of enrichment" (2). Jane Donawerth also observes the need for "broader definitions of rhetoric" that include a female aesthetic of communication (xv). Women's rhetoric has at times sidestepped established analytical theories and instead used previously unsanctioned methods to attract audiences directly.

Nineteenth-century women developed discursive strategies to fit podium, pulpit, stage, and page. They honed speaking voices in the service of such specific movements as women's rights, abolition, and temperance, testing and adopting tactics that resonated with listeners. Speakers for these movements shaped the nation in no small part, engendering fresh praxes of communication used by advocates for both community and national causes. As they rallied for the public good, female speakers and writers engaged with multiple social causes, their words patterning a country's identity and body politic. Women reformers often did not limit themselves to a single issue, the rhetoric from different movements thereby becoming interlinked and strengthened. Speakers and writers attended to each other's words to develop tactics interactively. Temperance proponents, for example, showed the influence of speakers who "argued for women's rights while overtly supporting the temperance cause" (Mattingly 15).[19] Similarly, women's rights proponents reflected the methods of abolitionists, as when Margaret Fuller admired antislavery speakers, who could "subdue the prejudices of their hearers" (quoted in Kolodny 142). Moreover, female abolitionists mirrored the use of deflection employed by temperance reformers, enabling them to broach an issue thought to be "inappropriate" or "unfeminine" for a woman speaker.[20] Many techniques for persuading audiences were tried in one venue then modeled and refined in another, so that the combined issues of temperance, women's rights, and abolition formed a seedbed to yield different rhetorical tactics to urge changes that would benefit the public welfare. Women reformers improved tactics of communication through the cross-pollination of different causes' rhetoric.

Regardless of gender, nineteenth-century citizenry took rhetoric seriously as a practice that kept democracy vital, requiring it as part of educational curricula to be taught to both boys and girls. Its importance stemmed from the national conviction that to build a robust republic with healthy civic institutions, each American must know how to speak effectively. As Johnson observes, nineteenth-century rhetoric was defined as "the art that contributed" to the "workings of the political process, the disposition of justice, and the maintenance of the public welfare and social conscience" (139). Women's contributions to this rhetoric carried the onus of exemplifying a feminine moral virtue that would bolster the republic by offering moral uplift. Cheree Carlson describes a situation in which there existed a heightened American "fascination with the 'proper' female character, for as she went, so, symbolically, went the national character" (5). Female speakers advanced discourse to persuade the public of the need for civic service, at the same time that they fulfilled the ideal of gendered service that would fortify the nation's virtue.

Perhaps the first thing to say about the nineteenth-century art of persuasion is that a woman's discourse of "persuasion," per se, did not exist—at least not in the way the word is traditionally understood. If persuasion designates the act of attempting to exhort a listener to change her or his conceptions, then female discursive practice remains an uneasy fit, because women typically aimed to draw audiences into conversation. Rather than "win" the point, they attempted to *win over* the listener, so to speak. Many historians stress the lack of *agon* in female rhetoric and the plethora of communications that were dialogic. Indeed, Donawerth asserts that many women speakers claimed conversation as their rhetorical model, but that only a single male theorist did so (344).

Not confrontational but rather engaging, women aimed for interchange, as for example in the conversational style Margaret Fuller and Sarah Josepha Hale embraced. Fuller famously used conversation in place of argumentation to win support for women's rights causes, eschewing "the authoritarianism of coercion and the manipulative strategies of the disempowered, endeavoring instead to create a collaborative process" (Kolodny 159). Fuller aimed for shared conversation with her audience, enjoying repartee and the exchange of ideas in a comfortable venue that could build community. Likewise, Sarah Josepha Hale, editor of *Godey's Lady's Book*, used conversation as a tactic and even a metaphor, to the extent that she "invited her readers to participate with her in constructing the magazine" (Tonkovich 155). In effect, Hale solicited readers to weigh in on the magazine's projects, building consensus and constructing an audience of likeminded reformers with "similar assumptions and concerns," which she sometimes mobilized to take "concerted political action" (Tonkovich 167).

Women tended to employ discourse that sparked affinity, a tactic Mattingly refers to in her study of temperance rhetoric as the use of "comfortable" and "familiar" speech, and what Jacqueline Bacon calls, in her study of abolitionist rhetoric, the strategies of indirection and deflection. Notably, as Bacon shows, women abolitionists used these rhetorical tactics of indirection and deflection in some of the following ways: the presentation of an argument as "queries to her audience" (159), the seeming disclaimer of judgment while actually arguing a point (160), the discussion of "an 'unfeminine' topic while professing to avoid it" (161), and the removal of herself from the argument by using a persona so as to "employ strategies such as irony and attack" (162). Such a conversational model invited involvement, pluralism, and a dynamism between speaker and audience. Bacon's insightful discussion of the abolitionist tactics of indirection and deflection will be called on often in the fol-

lowing pages of this study to show how nurse narrators employed discourse. Nurses shaped memoirs not to challenge or intimidate, but to include and rally—the goal being not to shut down a resisting audience but to precipitate questions, the seeds of which might germinate into later realizations.

NURSE NARRATIVE STRATEGIES arose within the larger history of nineteenth-century rhetoric developed to advocate for cultural movements in the decades directly preceding the 1860s. I must offer the caveat that I advance narrative strategies not for the sake of developing a history of rhetoric but use the tools of rhetoric to situate the narratives and thereby view more lucidly how nurses represented themselves. My intellectual goal remains that of contextualizing the nurse memoir through rhetorical history, but even more that of scrutinizing the memoirist's modes of expression page by page, in the rich experience of reception that any individual reader owns as she or he grapples with a text. Given that the nurse memoir initiates a subgenre of literature, the idiosyncrasies of narrative expression prove worth tracking for their comprehensive communication patterns.

While Civil War nurse narrators used discourse that was representative of the social movements of their times and singular to their gender, they also spoke to the exigencies of their personal situations as they performed relief work in difficult hospital or camp environments. The most crucial and pervasive nurse-narrative strategy, commensurate with the intent of nineteenth-century women's rhetoric in general, was the use of conversation. Like other women reform speakers, the nurse memoirist employed a conversational rhetoric to establish an inclusive tone and vital sense of exchange with her audience, which engendered a protracted writer–reader bond, allowing her to recount, sometimes in necessarily disturbing detail, her experience. The goal of this intense relationship was to garner reader validation; indeed, the mid-century nurse narrator may have had an even more immediate, almost visceral, need to gain audience approval more quickly than did other women speakers, given the notoriety of female nursing. To comprehend the nurse's uphill narrative task, it is necessary for us to credit the female nurse's early battle with public reception, since the citizenry at large perceived that women working in hospitals risked becoming sexually dissolute.[21] Female nursing carried the stigma of sexual compromise, because in the past the job of nursing had been considered unfit for middle-class women; specifically, it included attending to partially nude men. In the attempt to quell public disapproval and protect against criticism, the memoirist projected instead scenes of integrity. Having chosen a potentially treacherous path of employment, the female nurse developed the rhetoric of conversation to avert social disapprobation, setting up a clear, confiding tone in order to win trust from her reader.

At the beginning of the war the female nurse did not have a ready audience for an account of her work because the public was of many minds—sometimes scandalized, sometimes curious, and also sometimes supportive. She struggled to demonstrate female probity at the same time that she appealed to readers at home who yearned for details of the war effort as they awaited word from the front about their own loved ones. With the onus on the narrator to protect her honor, she defended her choice of employment by recounting the story of each patient with tenderness and, if possible, she told an exciting tale as well. Using a rhetoric of conversation she reached readers anxious to hear descriptions of soldiers' medical treatment, functioning for her readers as a reliable witness, a first-person recorder, and a stand-in as a "protagonist" as well. She built an understated platform of conversation, showing that she identified with the reader even as she indicted and reshaped the cultural prescriptions assigned to women. The nurse generated confidence through the informal, even personal nature of the dynamic between author and audience. She nurtured firm ties with her audience, which we see, for example, in Alcott's sustained attempts at charm, Woolsey's supplications for specific soldier provisions, and Dunlap's use of a narrative stand-ins for the reader.[22] The primary narrative strategy the nurse narrator used was that of creating and galvanizing a narrator–audience bond, especially by recourse to a conversational apparatus—all other narrative strategies were more or less subsidiary to that.

Each narrator's sense of audience bond indexed the circulation of her text; that is to say, the writer-to-reader passage can be tracked, to an extent, by the marketing used to distribute her memoir for reader consumption. For example, Wheelock's narrative was sold by subscription. Local papers announced specific times when agents could make themselves available to peddle the work, a type of circulation that suggests a popular audience. Woolsey's narrative was supervised by the Sanitary Commission, and newspaper notices ensured that her writing was disseminated for free when a reader simply supplied an address. Sophronia Bucklin on at least some occasions sold volumes of her book outright and probably came into contact personally with readers. Such methods of distribution, along with newspaper reviews (which will be sampled in the following chapters) reveal a gestalt of the nurse's relationship with her audience.

While the aim of creating a reader bond took precedence, other distinct narrative strategies operated to work variations on that bond, as follows: tonal immediacy, maternal stance, and scenes of travel. One other, more rare, feature may or may not be seen as a narrative strategy: the nurse's interrogation of suffering as a corrective for the nation. For each nurse, strategies were cultivated and altered according to her temperament and the differing particulars of her service.

The narrative strategy of tonal immediacy conveyed the precipitate treatment that nurses gave soldiers in order to save their lives. Tonal immediacy is allied with the above-mentioned rhetorical tactics of deflection and indirection, which include the discussion of "an 'unfeminine' topic while professing to avoid it" (Bacon 161). The strategy of tonal immediacy added a rushed narrative tempo. Once immersed in a memoir that proceeded at the lively speed of daily hospital life, the reader had no leisure to object to perceived infringements of decorum. The nurse narrator adopted the tone of plain talk, delivered in hurried, dashed-off segments, as the epigraph to this chapter by Julia Dunlap demonstrates: "These notes were jotted down as the incidents occurred" (xiii). Julia Wheelock, too, modeled the informal, animated tone when she stated, "I often sat upon a box or some rude bench, and held my book on my lap as I wrote" (v). Anna Morris Holstein, further, identified her narrative as "this simple story of hospital scenes, and the unpretending sketches" that are "arranged from the meager notes which were hurriedly written from the time they occurred" (v). Similarly, Elvira Powers stipulated that she did not mean for her book to function as an overview of the nurse's experience, but as "a simple record of scenes and events, just as they occurred from day to day under her own observations" (vi). This diction is nothing if not off the cuff and on the pulse.

The immediacy claimed for the prose, however, is for the most part tonal rather than actual, for however much narrators chronicled their experience in diaries or letters, they later revised those notes toward their finished composition. In other words, the narrator typically recorded the private, raw scenes that cut to the experience at hand during the grip of events, then kept the intonation of diaristic flurry when composing the finished work. Most narrators performed a somewhat extraordinary conversion from private to public expression, which transmitted faith in women's ability to retain their poise under fire, so to speak, and create a narrator-protagonist who made a valid contribution to the national project.[23] The language used in their book titles indicates the authors' preference for spontaneity: *Sketches, Three Weeks, Notes, Pencillings.* Tonal immediacy reflected the experience of shuffled assignments, impermanent locales, instantaneous attendance on incoming wounded, abrupt reversals in orders, and patient relationships characterized by sudden loss. In this environment the narrator observed swift cuts of action, writing a kind of precursor to more contemporary, wartime journalism that features spur-of-the-moment accounts.[24] Later, the nurse distilled the story while retaining the precipitate diction.[25]

The maternal stance was also born of indirection and deflection and a subsidiary of the writer–reader conversational bond, as well. The maternal stance was created or suggested by the nurse narrator to allay audience fears of impropriety in their interactions with soldiers. By ensconcing military medicine within the boundaries of home medicine, the nurse cribbed from Florence Nightingale the power of the mother to help her win the hearts of readers, as many cultural historians have pointed out. Silber, for instance, states that the perspective of mother "allowed women to envision a national community that was more like a broad, extended family than a socially stratified and ethnically divided society" (*Daughters* 202). The maternal gesture allowed the nurse to tend to patients more comfortably, negotiate with surgeons more effectively, pitch herself as the domestic protector of her "boys," and cast the nation as family.

Pointing out the rhetorical value for political reformers in positioning themselves as mother, Johnson analyzes Theodore Tilton's 1869 biographical construction of Elizabeth Cady Stanton in *Eminent Women of the Age*; Tilton justifies Stanton's "rhetorical activism" by rendering her an "idealized mother figure," one who was "not a woman out of place on the podium but rather a woman doing exactly what she should be doing, mothering the nation with her words of truth and concern" (*Gender* 137). Johnson also shows Elizabeth Stuart Phelps enacting a similar rhetorical gesture in 1884 when writing a biography about Mary Livermore, a journalist, women's rights advocate, and Civil War nurse. Phelps described Livermore as a woman "'who mothered half the land'" (113). As an aside, Johnson wonders if the maternal posture in general was actually a strategy or simply "an earnest articulation of a view of women that they [the biographers] actually believed" (116). As concerns the nurse narrators, who were using the maternal posture before these instances, their articulation was certainly a strategy. Whereas Stanton and Livermore were both biological mothers before and during the war, most of the nurse narrators were not mothers when they wrote their memoirs, so that choosing a maternal stance for them was clearly crafted and strategic.[26]

Through this important maternal stance, nurses attended wounded soldiers at bedsides, including soldiers who were fatally wounded, some of whom they helped to face death. Drew Gilpin Faust defines the nineteenth-century "Good Death" as a passing away that included the presence of a circle of family and friends, and contends that, given the mass fatalities in the Civil War, such a good death was rarely experienced (6). If a patient was able to approximate a good death, though, it was in many instances under the aegis of a nurse who eased his last hours and facilitated the process by acting as provisional mother. Aiding a soldier in this way, indispensible to his comfort, the narrator subtly demonstrated women's nursing expertise as she made possible the honorable decease of a patient. Along the way she fortified a relationship with readers as well.

An iteration of the maternal stance is the populist maternal stance, a position that highlighted the brace of affinity shared by female nurses and working-class soldiers. Both nurses and working-class soldiers implicitly understood their labor conditions to be similar, as they took marching orders from commanding officers and developed a rapport through shared hardship.[27] Narrators showed scenes of trust and camaraderie between nurses and army privates in a variety of ways, in many of which women pushed the boundaries of red tape or blurred the lines of regulations so as to help procure food, supplies, and services the soldiers needed. As the voice of the populist mother-of-the-ward, the nurse aligned herself with the rank-and-file soldier in patriotic loyalty. She came into her own by taking on the role of mother so that she could minister more efficiently and directly to her soldier–sons and embody the vital potential of America's future as a family.

When the memoirist detailed the scene of travel, especially travel on the initial route to the hospital, she highlighted the nurse's sacrifice with another tactic; once again, the tactic forms a subsidiary of the conversational bond summoned to instill trust in the reader. Narrators depicted initial motivations for joining up and initial modes of travel for women nurses journeying far from home, often for the first time in their lives. Nurses undertook difficult and uncertain transport arrangements, meeting up with strangers, and arriving at forbidding hospitals or camps. Many readers would have registered empathy for these relief workers as they weathered such discomfort and anxiety. Narrators extended themselves to their audience by creating parallels between warfront and homefront, adding an element of adventure to these travel descriptions to pique readers' imagination and to foster their admiration. Concerning the hardships endured and feats accomplished, memoirs by Alcott, Powers, Holstein, and Wheelock made dramatic use of travel as a narrative strategy.

Finally, a more unusual but no less important feature of the nurse narrative is the speaker's interrogation of the validity of suffering as a corrective for the nation. The feature of interrogating suffering incorporates a potentially dangerous eclipse of the rhetoric of patriotism, even sometimes to the point of elision. At rare but notable impasses, the nurse questioned affliction as a national project, and did so more clearly in the later narratives, particularly those of Powers, Holstein, and Wheelock. Acting as interlocutor, the female nurse on the one hand pleaded patriotically for justice for the soldier in terms of supplies and care, but on the other experienced an occasional break in narrative voice that risked breaking with patriotic discourse. The points at which nurse rhetoric evidences a crack—even a hairline crack—provide a discontinuity fascinating for the fact that the nurse narrative stands so carefully crafted at most times—and yet, these are the points, albeit laconic, at which she is most directly in conversation with her readers. Probably only by identifying so thoroughly with her audience could she have managed this difficult operation. Some nurses, encountering pain and death on a daily basis, experienced caregiver's trauma, and to the extent that she was exposed to unrelenting suffering on a large scale, she could come to seem detached from meaning. Certainly nurses experienced less physical pain than their soldier–patients (except when contracting disease), but they felt their own strain of psychological anguish in witnessing the continual suffering of unnumbered wounded and sick patients. At times nurses voiced the absence of meaning they had registered in the midst of such misery.

The nurse's attempt to articulate such trauma revealed occasional dissociations in language as she struggled with fractures in representation that resulted from the difficulty of assigning meaning to pain. At times she used prose less as a matter of composition than decomposition, so to speak, conveying a foundering reality in the face of prevailing illness and lack of wholeness, writing in the attempt to patch together something that seemed incapable of being reunited.[28] In contradistinction to patriotic memoirs that foregrounded cultural myths of the ineffable American spirit, written to subdue war stress, the nurse narrator at uncommon junctures disarticulated those myths to reveal an unthinkable, inscrutable gap or rent in the national psyche in which pain remained unredeemed. Only in flashes did she broach these moments of doubt about the American project of war, expressing psychological dislocations of her own, mirroring the displaced body of the wounded soldier. These disarticulations occurred in glimpses as the nurse strove to uphold duty and worked in hospital wards that could seem to turn at any moment into a fragile facade, ready to collapse, as she sometimes felt it, on the death of a single patient.

THE SEVEN MEMOIRS in *Civil War Nurse Narratives*, arranged chronologically, all focus intensively on the narrative strategies that construct and strengthen the rhetoric of the writer–reader conversational bond. The first chapter, "Louisa May Alcott's *Hospital Sketches*," examines Alcott's hands-on conversation with her readers by demonstrating that she initiated the bond with the reader early on, when segments of her narrative appeared in the Boston newspaper, *The Commonwealth*, and she developed it further when she composed the published book version. One major benefit of this new analysis of *Hospital Sketches* is that Alcott can be understood more comprehensively in the context of the nurse narrative subgenre of war literature. "Georgeanna Woolsey's *Three Weeks at Gettysburg*," the second chapter, determines how Woolsey established the rhetoric of conversation by affiliating with readers whom she inspired to donate supplies to the United States Sanitary Commission. Working to connect narrator and audience, she used the through-line of linkage to prompt consideration of other connections as well, such as those between black and white workers and between Northern and Southern soldiers. The third chapter, "Julia Dunlap's *Notes of Hospital Life*," corroborates the identity of Julia Dunlap, anonymous until 2010, through her work at the Philadelphia Hospital of the Protestant Episcopal Church, and verifies her target audience, at least initially, as that of the members of the church who sponsored the hospital. Dunlap championed the working-class soldier and framed her project as a venture in Christian benevolence and sympathy, a framing that was sometimes uneasy and subject to revision.

Following the savvy Powers on her wide-ranging journeys, "Elvira Powers's *Hospital Pencillings*" demonstrates how she used the narrative strategy of travel to establish a connection with her reader. She registered more dissent in the workplace than narrators before her, buttressing her dissent by adopting the rhetoric of women's rights, abolitionism, New England civil disobedience, and American patriotism. Anna Morris Holstein's *Three Years in Field Hospitals of the Army of the Potomac*" covered Holstein's fieldwork during and after some of the most wrenching campaigns of the Civil War. Holstein provided the most extensive example of the narrative strategy of interrogating the validity of suffering as a corrective for the nation, engaging the last half or so of the book in a running meditation on the meaning of death in war; because she saw and represented mass affliction, she needed an especially strong conversational connection with her readers.

The chapter, "Sophronia Bucklin's *In Hospital and Camp*," argues that Bucklin spoke primarily from the vantage of women's rights rhetoric to build an affinity with her reader and to justify dissent. She forged a bond with the rank-and-file soldier, gradually coming to work alongside black soldiers and black women relief workers as she discovered her own disturbing assumption of white privilege. Finally, a kind of showcase for how a nurse narrator could fashion her book is offered in "Julia Wheelock's *The Boys in White*." Access to Wheelock's papers permits an investigation of the tactical choices in diction she used to promote reader reception. Wheelock pursued fair treatment for patients in the greater Washington, DC area where she labored and sometimes disagreed with hospital authorities over administrative decisions. Threading the motif of "the boys in white" throughout her memoir, she charted the nature of grief on individual and national levels.

ANY MILITARY CONFLICT brings about major social shifts, accompanied by fluctuations in modes of representation: "Wars have always been profoundly connected to subversion in the representation of functions of gender and changes in the use of literary genres" (Usandizaga ix). To some extent the female Civil War nurse participated in this "subversion in the representation" of both gender and genre when she wrote her memoir, an alternative representation that satisfied the need for a vibrant American literature during the war years. The nurse narrative formed a worthy subgenre of war literature that recorded the lived ideology of women's rights even as it revalued social struggles during the nation's most cataclysmic event. The narrative, as Homi Bhabha attests, remains not only a literary product but an active agent: "To study the nation through its narrative address does not merely draw attention to its language and rhetoric; it also attempts to alter the conceptual object itself" (*Nation* 3). In the course of rapidly shifting events, the nurse narrator, within the context of her new vocation, counterpoised domestic values and public obligations, altering the conceptual object of America as a gendered work in progress.

She addressed her memoir to a particular generation of women steeped in social movements and the rhetoric of those movements, such as women's rights, abolition, benevolence, and temperance. She cultivated an audience by way of these perspectives and the discourses they used, creating her own conversational apparatus to attract an audience. Her readers studied the nation in part through women's personal and individual addresses. Through the narrative the nurse conceived a fresh female citizen who defined herself by action, at the same time exemplifying a praxis by which a woman could speak of practical, social, and moral concerns of import for the country. In recording those struggles the memoir refigured, to some degree, the significance of the war itself. The nurse narrator framed issues from a point of view distinct from the historical accounts of soldiers or statesmen and inscribed the concerns of that decade from the perspective of a gender not heard from often enough in histories of the Civil War.

Certainly, nothing was set down in malice . . . (73)

CHAPTER ONE

Louisa May Alcott's *Hospital Sketches*

A Readership

Alcott was taken aback by the success of *Hospital Sketches*. A group of notes tossed off in a couple of months after she returned from hospital service, the book was hardly the work she would have envisioned for significant acceptance by a readership. The editors of *The Commonwealth*, a Boston newspaper, had suggested she arrange and submit the letters she wrote during her Civil War nursing service, and she recorded in her April 1863 journal that they "thought them witty & pathetic, I didn't, but I wanted money so I made three 'Hospital Sketches'" (*Journals* 118). *The Commonwealth* editors found her letters remarkable, but Alcott's curt phrase, "I didn't," spoke volumes for her own opinion. Nonetheless, she promptly adapted and revised the correspondence she had written home a few months earlier while serving at the Union Hotel Hospital in Washington, DC (she said she wrote three of these "Hospital Sketches," above, but she eventually penned four altogether). The four writings were published by

The Commonwealth as "Hospital Sketches I," through "Hospital Sketches IV," appearing from May through June of 1863.[1] Soon after the columns appeared, in August of the same year, James Redpath published Alcott's book, in which she heavily revised those four columns. She also added two new chapters, the first two of the book: "Obtaining Supplies" and "A Forward Movement." The newspaper pieces and the book both received immediate attention, but Alcott was confounded by it, as she wrote on November 6, 1863, to a friend of the family, Mary Elizabeth Waterman: "'Hospital Sketches' still continues a great joke to me, & a sort of perpetual surprise-party, for to this day I cannot see why people like a few extracts from topsey turvey letters written on inverted tin kettles, in my pantry, while waiting for gruel to warm or poultices to cool, for boys to wake and be tormented, on stairs, in window seats & other sequestered spots favorable to literary inspiration" (*Letters* 95).

Louisa May Alcott, daughter of Transcendentalist teacher and writer Amos Bronson Alcott, didn't publish her famous novel *Little Women* until 1868, a half-decade after *Hospital Sketches*, which was based on her service at the Union Hotel Hospital in Washington, DC, where she nursed the incoming wounded from the disastrous Battle of Fredericksburg during December 1862. *Hospital Sketches* launched Alcott's career, and the composition of it showed her a way to cultivate a narrative brio and a means to establish a close bond with an audience. Alcott herself acknowledged that the book "never made much money, but showed me 'my style'" (*Journals* 124); in other words, though it didn't make her wealthy, it did light an aesthetic that guided her subsequent literary productions. The development of Alcott's style forms a primary concern in this chapter, wherein her attention to her readers can be tracked by way of her revisions, which focus on a conversational bonding. Having struggled as a writer before the release of her newspaper pieces, Alcott suddenly found the literary world taking notice, with her work reaching an audience broad enough to garner some acclaim. She learned quickly from this reception and revised *The Commonwealth* pieces, basing the publication of her book on a rhetoric tailored to the reader.

Alcott chronicled the reception of *The Commonwealth* contributions in her journal the same month the serial ended, noting that she was both

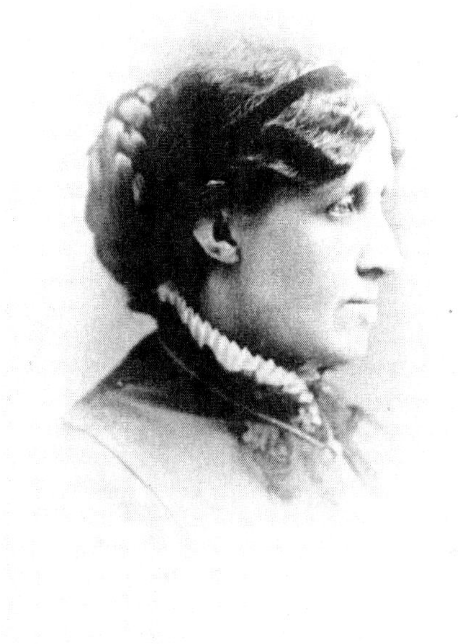

Louisa May Alcott, 1862–1863

MOLLUS Massachusetts Civil War Photographs, United States Army Heritage and Education Center, Carlisle, PA

surprised and encouraged by "the commendation bestowed" upon these pieces, "which were noticed, talked & inquired about much to my surprise & delight" (119). Upon publication of the book in August, though, she recorded uncertainty, confiding that the sketches "keep on making friends for me, though I dont [*sic*] get used to the thing at all & think it must be all a mistake" (120).[2] It is touching to see Alcott dumbfounded by recognition; she told Redpath on August 28, the month of the book's publication, "such a burst of new plans & projects rather made my head spin" (88). By September, Redpath was planning another edition of the book, and in October Alcott found herself still disbelieving: "If ever there was an astonished young woman it is myself, for things have gone on so swimmingly of late I dont know who I am. A year ago I had no publisher & went begging with my wares, now *three* have asked me for something" (121). The success astonished her to the point that she felt her identity shifting, as when she wrote, above, "I dont know who I am." She was confounded probably less because of a lack of artistic self-confidence than because of a bewilderment that it was this particular book—a realistic blend of fact and fiction, instead of a story of sensation—that provided a career breakthrough. In a kind of journal summary for the year of 1863, she wrote almost poignantly, "Hospital Sketches come out & I find I've done a good thing without knowing it" (122).

Alcott received positive responses from both the smaller circle of her townspeople and the larger circle of national readers and critics. She expressed delight at the warm reception from residents of her home village of Concord: "I have the satisfaction of seeing my towns folk buying, reading, laughing & crying over it wherever I go" (*Letters* 88). From a slightly larger circle she also took pleasure in the observations of an army surgeon who visited Concord to inform her that he found her characterization of army mules to be particularly true-to-life; she wrote with humor that the surgeon "considered my mules striking likenesses" (88). As regards the larger, national circle, *Hospital Sketches* became known to the extent that in at least one case, a nurse read aloud to soldiers from Alcott's book, which they enjoyed.[3] Critically, *Hospital Sketches* garnered several good reviews, among them one in 1863 calling her work "not only remarkable but memorable," lauding the presence of cultivated women nurses in war hospitals, so that "we have prepared the way for a new variety of literature which will still further open our sympathies for the sick and wounded soldiers" (Clark 12). Notably, the reviewer used class stereotypes to mark the presence of female nurses as respectable, but in addition saw the possibility of the female nurse writing "a new variety of literature," a prescient claim in the light of the books written by nurses that appeared after Alcott's book.

It must be said at the outset that Alcott's narrative is not, strictly speaking, a narrative. She was circumspect about nonfiction and covered her wariness with Dickensian aplomb. She developed her text to involve a quirky, likeable, and at times slightly exasperating narrator whose convictions were tested by rapid-fire incidents. *Hospital Sketches* was "thinly fictionalized," according to Elizabeth Young (73), and Alcott fictionalized it for a reason, fearing that the unadorned memoir would reveal and overexpose the narrator—that is, herself.[4] Elbert notes that Alcott was "troubled" by the publication of *Hospital Sketches*, feeling vulnerable as a narrator who had "previously hidden behind pseudonyms" (164). In

light of her desire to endear herself to her audience, she may have been anxious to screen some of her more potentially objectionable opinions. Hence, she created a narrator who tried to ingratiate herself to readers, hoping to beguile them into accepting the uncommon world she inhabited at the Union Hotel Hospital where women nurses, controversial at the time, labored.

This chapter examines how Alcott carefully established reader rapport, from the epigraph on the book's front cover to "A Postscript" at the end.[5] In the cover epigraph she voiced her concern with pleasing the audience so that "'no offence could be took,'" and in "A Postscript" on the last page she expressed her desire to attend to the "cheerfulnesses" of the nurse's existence. However, as we shall see, Alcott counterweighed the "cheerfulnesses" with the inevitable "dismals" that occasionally surfaced despite her conscious efforts. Finally, Alcott, a staunch abolitionist, recorded some nonetheless unsettling interactions with black hospital workers, and the attempt to ameliorate the political aims of abolition with the new need for social equality in everyday life also became part of her mediation with the reader. *Hospital Sketches* exhibits fault lines that trace where Alcott used her letters and journals as raw drafts from which she composed a finished newspaper account, then afterwards a yet more polished book.

The Cheerfulnesses

The final chapter of *Hospital Sketches*, "A Postscript," reads a little like a contemporary media Q & A, with questions posed to the writer, and it clues us to the sensitive, even volatile, issues Alcott attempted to skirt in trying not to offend the reader. Some of the questions in "A Postscript" were asked outright by readers of *The Commonwealth* columns, and some questions can be extrapolated by looking at the "answers" she gave: Are there church services for the soldiers? Can friends and family come to nurse their loved ones in the wards? What domestic comforts does the military hospital offer? Do nurses have a choice as to whether to witness amputations? In brief, Alcott's readers wanted to know how the war hospital accommodated Christian faith, family, friends, domesticity, and women who might want to be nurses. Though she had answered many of the questions directly in the fourth of her four installments of "Hospital Sketches," she was unable to answer one.

This one, which she seemed very keen to address in the book, was posed by a reader who apparently had accused her of writing in a tone too lively for the columns' subject matter. The reader apparently asked whether Alcott's voice was appropriate for the material, finding her use of humor off-putting in the face of the enormity of Civil War casualties. Always concerned about reader reaction, Alcott must have felt particular consternation in singling out this one objection so prominently, but nonetheless stood firm. Interestingly, she defended her levity by drawing on the informal commendation of her companion laborers at the workplace, reporting that "since the appearance of these hasty Sketches, I have heard from several of my comrades at the Hospital; and their approval assures me that I have not let sympathy and fancy run away with me" (73). Alcott substantiated her fictionalized work, paradoxically, by deferring to her actual "comrades at the Hospital," people who shared the hospital experience and knew firsthand the graphic details of medical work.

She protected her style in *Hospital Sketches*, a deliberate mix of truth and invention—a type of writing she had developed expressly for the book. In this same paragraph about levity, she furthered her defense:

> Certainly, nothing was set down in malice, and to the serious-minded party who objected to a tone of levity in some portions of the Sketches, I can only say that it is a part of my religion to look well after the cheerfulnesses of life, and let the dismals shift for themselves. (73)

Managing the reader's concern, Alcott pronounced that she pursued an ongoing project of finding optimism in the business of living, keeping abjection and melancholy outside her purview. The strategy of attending to the cheerfulnesses in *Hospital Sketches* made for the prominence of a sanguine tone, in keeping with her claim that such was part of her "religion." She fostered the cheerfulnesses with heartening and witty prose. Though she responded only to this one reader who had taken issue with her tone, she was most likely anxious about disapproval, especially because the two new chapters she added to the four newspaper installments to comprise the book were even more chipper. She weighed in on the project of cultivating a writing style characterized by an off-the-cuff optimism and relentless alacrity: "As no two persons see the same thing with the same eyes, my view of hospital life must be taken through my glass and held for what it is worth" (73). Not surprisingly, in the early pages of the book she identified the "glass" of her main character, Tribulation Periwinkle, as rosy, when she described the Periwinkle family as wearing "rose-colored spectacles" (4). The irrepressible Alcott cheer was to become a signature force for her as an author.

In these beginning chapters, "Obtaining Supplies" and "A Forward Movement," Alcott initiated the nurse-narrative strategy of describing the nurse's travel, a tactic that performed the service of cushioning the perceptions of detractors who might initially have surmised that nurse working conditions were morally compromising.[6] The scene of travel was often preceded by a statement of the nurse's motivation for serving in the hospital, as in the very first sentence of *Hospital Sketches*, when Tribulation unabashedly proclaimed to her family, "'I want something to do'" (3). She addressed the sentence "to no one in general," so as to include her whole family—and by extension her whole readership—in the process of mulling over the problem: a woman wants something to do, wants to occupy herself with a meaningful project. The family responded in kind, her father suggesting that she write a book, her mother that she teach, her sister that she take a husband, and another sister that she act on the stage. In proposing teaching and taking a husband as choices, her family proffered options that would have been in accordance with customary expectations for nineteenth-century women, with the option of writing a book also acceptable.[7] The family suggested civilian choices, despite the fact that the country's conflict had begun to turn into the most devastating war in United States history—until Tribulation's brother offered the alternative she needed: "Go nurse the soldiers." To this she replied concisely, "I will!" (3). The suggestion, framed by the voice of her brother, gave Tribulation the license to move into this new arena where women performed work for a military cause, and her jaunty response may have been designed to cue readers to respond in kind.

Alcott scuttled possible public censure of women nurses by enticing the reader with an exuberant statement of the motivation of her protagonist, Tribulation Periwinkle, her brother's suggestion, and the ensuing enthusiasm of her family. Upon making her flash decision, the family became involved in imagining the specifics of her new vocation, working variations on each other's ideas. As the Periwinkles were "a hopeful race," their imaginings served to "set the whole family in a blaze of enthusiasm" (4), as they constructed an invented institution:

> A model hospital was erected, and each member had accepted an honorable post therein. The paternal P. was chaplain, the maternal P. was matron, and all the youthful P.s filled the pod of futurity with achievements whose brilliancy eclipsed the glories of the present and the past. Arriving at this satisfactory conclusion, the meeting adjourned, and the fact that Miss Tribulation was available as an army nurse went abroad on the wings of the wind. (4)

The family built a domestic idyll of the war hospital, including father, mother, "and all the youthful P.s," transposing familial closeness onto the site of the war workplace in an image custom-made for an audience that cherished home relationships.

This segment clearly shows Alcott reaching out to her readership by involving the family in the national project of service to the Union. In some ways the Periwinkle family anticipated the similar imaginative energy of the more famous March family of Alcott's 1868 *Little Women*, both groups distanced from the extreme eccentricity of the actual Alcotts while keeping the heartwarming quirks.[8] Alcott drew a verbal picture of the Periwinkle family crest, including roosters that wore "rose-colored spectacles, and are lineal descendants of the inventor of aerial architecture" (3–4).[9] Having made her decision, Tribulation exhibited an alacrity that in turn stoked the reader's enthusiasm.

To intensify reader reception, Alcott transposed the domestic life of her family onto the imagined life of the military, as the Periwinkles did by imagining themselves to be personnel in a war hospital. Tribulation designated her future post in every particular, coopting the language of regimented life to describe her existence, while still residing at home:

"I turned military at once, called my dinner my rations, saluted all new comers, and ordered a dress parade that very afternoon" (4). She used army diction to pun on actions carried out domestically, referring to the chore of airing laundry on a fence as "picket duty." She also called the work of mending apparel the act of attending "weak and wounded" clothes to make them "ready for active service again" (5). Before ever seeing a soldier, Tribulation selected language to fuse home and battlefield, and drew the reader into the process of readying herself for hospital work.

Shouldering her civilian traveling bag, which she denominated her military "knapsack," Tribulation expressly requested the reader to allow this: "do let me preserve the unities" (5). In a conversational move she entreated the reader to permit preservation of the "unities," a reference to classic literary theory: the unities conventionally require that a work of literature have unity of action (plot), time (of short duration), and space (a single location). On the narrative level, Alcott's wish to preserve the unities was ironic, given that *Hospital Sketches* itself preserved none of these: the plot is scattershot, the time arches over a few chaotic months, and the space is a pastiche of locales including the family's Massachusetts home, the Washington, DC hospital, and scenes around the capital. In addition, the very genre of *Hospital Sketches* hardly preserves the unities, mixed as it is between fiction and nonfiction. Alcott inculcated this small but incisive pun into her dramatization of the female nurse sallying forth to help the Northern cause, and though she joked and pleaded with her audience to "let" her preserve the unities in the face of her soon-to-be chaotic life, readers knew, on a more profound level, that they had no power to let anyone preserve the unities during wartime. A trenchant phrase, "preserving the unities" also referred, of course, to the much larger vision of Civil War politics, echoing the commonly voiced Northern rallying sentiment of "preserving" the Union.

Tribulation's final act of leave-taking from home occurred in a terse interchange with her mother, colored by her mother's patriotic courage as she relinquished her child. Reflecting many contemporaneous depictions of the male soldier leaving home, in which the mother is called on to sacrifice her child for the larger cause, Alcott reanimated the scene with the gender twist that the mother was saying farewell to her daughter. In this way Alcott validated the action of the female worker leaving to serve her country. Tribulation, recognizing the emotional difficulty, said she would stay if her mother requested it, and her mother answered immediately, "But I don't; go, and the Lord will take care of you" (5). Alcott's journals suggest that she and her own mother played out nearly this exact scene, her mother saying, "No, go! and the Lord be with you!" (*Journals* 110). In assigning ultimate authority to her mother, Alcott invested her book with the cultural capital to support the women nurses contributing to that effort.

In a strange turn immediately afterward, however, Alcott used wedding imagery to depict Tribulation's departure by train: Trib gave "a blithe farewell as if going on a bridal tour—though I believe brides don't usually wear cavernous black bonnets and fuzzy brown coats" (6). Again, Alcott mixed domestic and warfront imagery when she said, "I confess that the head under the funereal coal-hood fermented with all manner of high thoughts and heroic purposes 'to do or die'—perhaps both" (6). Subtly elicited in the words, "I do," she offered the assent of a bride and conflated it in the military-minded phrase, "to do or die"—a phrase that recalls Tennyson's poem, "The Charge of the Light Brigade," which emphasized the importance of duty in the call to war. Apropos of Trib's circumstance, the words reveal an underlying fear that she was riding into the Valley of Death as she journeyed to a hospital where she would attend wounded and dying soldiers. Further, when she said, "at this juncture I took the veil," she indicated that she was now wedded to her new vocation of military devotion. Movingly, though, she used the veil, too, to find a way to do some private crying, relating that, "what I did behind it [the veil] is nobody's business," thereby marking the action of wearing the veil as female behavior. She surprised the reader once more, however, by paralleling her experience with that of the "best" and "bravest" male soldier, whom she described as precisely the one "who cries when his mother says 'Good-bye'" (6).

Alcott encompassed both military and domestic realms by using puns that appeared jocular but registered a sense of foreboding, as for example in mingling wedding and funeral imagery. The American Civil War hospital, a consummately chaotic domain, was approached by the new female nurse, and Alcott accordingly expressed the ambiguity that a "topsy-turvy Trib" (6), reporting for duty, would have registered. She validated the nurse's sense of purpose, imbuing it with the commitment of both the new bride and the soldier, female and male, who set out to "do," which was Tribulation's concern on the very first page, when she exclaimed to her family, "I want something to do."

On first reading *Hospital Sketches*, we might wonder why it took Alcott so long to get Trib to the hospital, devoting as she did a good fourth of the text to a lengthy home description and travelogue before the character set foot inside a ward. The scenes of motivation, however, were sanctioned by family, and together with the scenes of travel, provided an absolutely necessary prelude to the book, formalizing the break in a woman's home experience before she took on the strange new duties of nurse. The travel to Washington, DC by train and boat proved arduous and shot through with bureaucratic tangles. Even the process of procuring tickets involved Tribulation's negotiation of a labyrinth of strange locations, as she "blundered into" an apartment "full of soldiers, surgeons, starers, and spittoons" (7). Despite the great comic value of such descriptions, this maze in fact featured inscrutable rules, taxing interactions, and impenetrable red tape, all of which called up reevaluations of the nurse's social and political position in her new work—and all of which Alcott used to involve the reader. Tribulation's discomfort was clear. For instance, not by nature being inclined to welcome male rescue, at one difficult juncture she spat out, "I'm a woman's rights woman" (9), but in this travel domain was willing to accept help from her brother-in-law, even though she would have refused it in ordinary times. In the midst of the melee Alcott encountered the need to defend herself from and simultaneously ingratiate herself to critics of women's rights who upheld women's dependence on men. Alcott established a conversational bond with her reader by allowing her audience to experience the rises and falls of this new venture. When Trib finally reached the "Hurly-Burly House," her name for the Union Hotel Hospital to which she'd been assigned, her heart beat faster, and she became fully aware of the reality of separation from her domestic circle: "it suddenly struck me that I was very far from home" (19).

Alcott continued to build audience involvement by showing Trib's first full day at the hospital, detailing her figurative and literal wake-up call when the wounded arrived from Fredericksburg, a conflict of particularly devastating loss for the Union. At this crux Trib again echoed the very first sentence of the book ("I want something to do"[1]), when she asked her hospital coworker about the incoming wounded, "What shall we have to do?" The coworker answered crisply, "'Wash, dress, feed, warm and nurse them for the next three months, I dare say'" (20). In this third chapter, labeled "One Day," Alcott described the grueling labor a nurse encountered during a twenty-four-hour period: tending to the grievously ill men from Fredericksburg, hurry, confusion, "the vilest odors," and the inevitable red tape that included the need for each wounded soldier to be "ticketed and registered" before he was provided with a bed. Tribulation more than once felt the need to weep, a feeling so strong she had to make sure it was "corked up" (22).

Maintaining a jaunty attitude, however, she fell back on her proclivity for punning, a means once more to articulate a synthesis between her previous family life and this regimented one, and here she lit on the felicitous word, "warfare." Seeming to revisit the laundry puns from the first chapter when she was at home, she reformulated them at work: "Having done up our human wash, and laid it out to dry, the second syllable of our version of the word 'war-fare' was enacted with much success" (26). The word "warfare," hence, melded war and home,[10] the home recalled in the "fare" of the bread, meat, soup, and coffee that was provided to the soldiers, but that also appeared on Trib's pinafore as it became splattered with the different foods. She claimed that she provided a sort of menu or "perambulating bill of fare, presenting samples of all the refreshments going or gone" (26). By way of such language play, Alcott evinced the jumbled nature of the hospital, where the opposites of hearth and field became intertwined in the female nurse's job. The difference between her punning at home and punning on the job was that the first depended on her act of imagining the new labor, and the second on the act of ac-

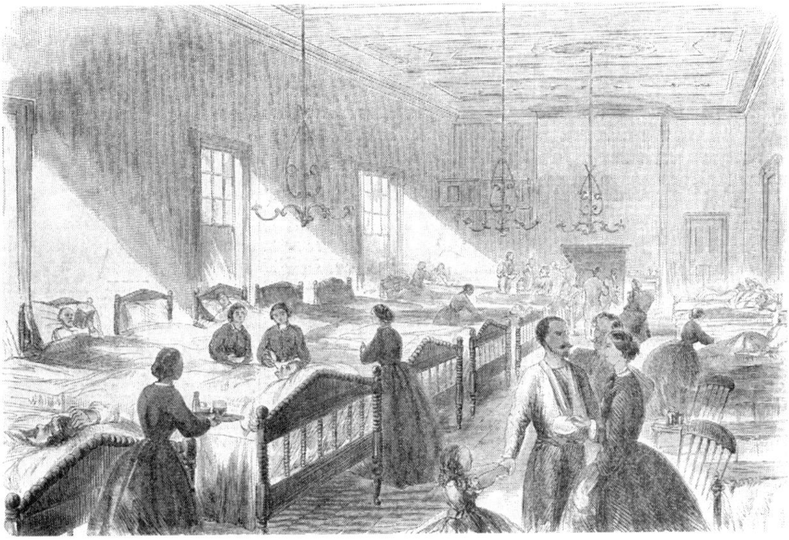

The United States Hospital at Georgetown, DC, called the Union Hotel Hospital

Schlesinger Library, Radcliffe Institute, Harvard University

cepting the difficult reality of it. She created a similar effect by calling attention to the word "ballroom," likewise a surreal conflation of civilian and military life, in that the Union Hotel Hospital "had been a hotel before hospitals were needed" (22), and one large room still kept the label of ballroom even as it housed a section of forty soldiers' beds: "my ward was in truth a *ball-room*, if gun-shot wounds could christen it" (22). Emphasizing both civilian and military realities, Alcott still struggled to preserve the unities.

She also attempted to normalize the workplace in a different way, introducing a kind of rite of initiation in the form of ritual ablution. One of the veteran nurses instructed Trib to begin washing patients, and Trib, scandalized and dumbfounded, responded: "If she had requested me to shave them all, or dance a horn-pipe on the stove funnel, I should have been less staggered; but to scrub some dozen lords of creation at a moment's notice, was really—really—" (23). Alcott hit the edge of the capacity for language to articulate her experience in this unfinished sentence, even as she steeled her audience for what would most alarm them—the female nurse's contact with the undressed male soldier's body. How she would resolve this problem would structure the future of her nursing career and the progress of her nurse narrative, too, given that she wished so adamantly to garner reader engagement. In order for Tribulation to wash her patients she had to face sexual anxiety and confute the social alarm that she was crossing entrenched gender lines.

The ritual washing included a metaphoric washing—or in her case, a metaphoric drowning, as she put it—in which she wet down her compunctions or "drowned my scruples in my washbowl" (23). Both soldier and nurse came clean as they crossed the gender barriers, Trib reporting that she "clutched my soap manfully" (23). She found a willing patient in the person of "a withered old Irishman, wounded in the head," who put her at ease to the point that the two of them ended up laughing "together." As they both trespassed the deeply inscribed cultural behaviors expected of gender, he was passive, because compromised by a wound, and she was active, having grabbed the domestically coded soap "manfully." Alcott enlarged the expected terms of the washing ritual to permit results for both her patient and herself, sanitizing them to ease the qualms of potentially uneasy readers who might have seen the nurse as jostling moral codes. She presented an ablution and the mutual cheer of the patient and nurse laughing together.

Alcott also eased potential misgivings by drawing on the narrative strategy of the populist maternal stance, the ritual of washing marking the infantilization of the weakened soldier. Tribulation functioned metaphorically as the mother who, in the process of washing the soldier, "scrubbed away like any tidy parent" (23). Just before this scrubbing, Trib experienced a felicitous vision of the relationship between nurse and patient in the countenance of the hospital matron, who stood in the ward among the ravaged bodies of soldiers arriving from Fredericksburg: "in the midst of it all, the matron's motherly face brought more comfort to many a poor soul, than the cordial draughts she administered, or the cheery words that welcomed all, making the hospital a home" (22). In this crucial tableau, the prototypical mother with beatific face centered the ward despite the frenzy surrounding her, and did so with equanimity.[11] To this example Trib aspired, claiming "a motherly affection for all" (32). She and other nurse narrators aspired, both as nurses and writers, to embody a serene maternal force in the midst of a hubbub and imbue an otherwise ghastly setting with tranquility, purpose, and cheer.[12]

Alcott controlled the narrative focus to conciliate her readers, coaxing them through her purposefully blithe tone to reframe their reception of the Civil War female nurse. Both the very end and the very beginning of *Hospital Sketches* revealed Alcott's special concern not to offend her readers and, in fact, to please and entertain them. If we have seen in the final chapter, "A Postscript," how she assured her audience that "nothing was set down in malice" (73), we will see how she avoided vexing her audience from the beginning of the book, attempting to endear herself before the reader even opened the cover. Alcott launched *Hospital Sketches* with a quirky drawing on the front that featured the unusual image of a fork, knife, and spoon joined in a triangle to frame a dinner plate.[13] At the center of the plate the illustrator inscribed the initials, "T. P."—mysterious to readers first encountering the book, but obvious if they had read the newspaper columns and met the main character, Tribulation Periwinkle. Just below the place setting, a whimsical epigraph emphasized her attention to audience: "'Which, naming no names, no offence could be took.'—Sairy [*sic*] Gamp."

This epigraph referred to Charles Dickens's 1843 novel, *Martin Chuzzlewit*, in the course of which the character Sarah Gamp, a nurse, claimed several times that she wished to give "no offence."[14] *Martin Chuzzlewit* affected a wide readership, for whom "the image of Sairey Gamp became the common stereotype of the unreformed, working-class nurse. Elderly, corpulent, disrespectful and predisposed to drunkenness, Sairey Gamp was at once a well-loved caricature and a universal representative of what needed to be driven out of the medical profession" (Judd 34). Alcott probably invoked the nurse to tease her audience and focus their attention on the stigmatization of the woman nurse, a kind of in-joke to promise readers that she would not repeat the misadventures of Sairey Gamp. By alluding to Gamp, Alcott signaled her commitment not to affront her audience by giving a verbal wink before the first page of *Hospital Sketches* was ever turned. She wished to alienate as few readers as possible, and several candidates for constituencies who might have taken umbrage existed: those who dismissed the idea of women nurses in military hospitals, recoiled at the cause of women's rights, bridled at Alcott's lack of conventional Christian doctrine, or disagreed with her spare but pointed criticism of the medical profession.[15] One can understand her reticence about writing nonfiction when one considers these many demographics of possible disapprobation in an era of roiling social change. In the attempt to endear herself to diverse readers, she created in Tribulation the anti-Gamp, the magnetic and rollicking character of Tribulation, with her relentless cheer.

By presenting the Dickens's epigraph, Alcott intimated that in the body of *Hospital Sketches* she would be, in Sarah Gamp's words, "naming no names," or at least would be obscuring real ones, in some cases creating fictionalized characters so as to render the memoir unobjectionable.[16] She used truncated monikers such as Dr. P. and Dr. Z. (a practice, of course, widespread in the nineteenth century) to ensure that no one with whom she worked was maligned.[17,18] Suggesting that her book as a whole retained historical authenticity, she nonetheless protected herself with a veneer of storytelling devices that included the omission of full names. Alcott described the narrative as "notes made by the way," similar to the claim in her letter, above, that the work consisted merely of "sketches," or tossed-off pieces, scribblings gathered together on inverted tin kettles, rather than a revised whole. She described her own particular blend of truth and fabrication in this way: "As travelers like to give their own impressions of a journey, though every inch of the way may have been described a half dozen times before, I add some of the notes made by the way, hoping that they will amuse the reader, and convince the skeptical that such a being as Nurse Periwinkle does exist, that she really did go to Washington, and that these Sketches are not romance" (12). In other words, she insisted that *Hospital Sketches* provided a genuine account—realism rather than romance—but, astonishingly, fixed that idea by claiming that her absurdly named character Tribulation Periwinkle really "does exist." In refusing to confess and identify herself as the protagonist, Alcott forwarded a distracting claim, a machination that goes to show how uneasy a mix her narrative was, and not least of all how much was at stake in creating the genre of the nurse narrative.

The strategy, by and large, paid off, as reviewers appreciated her cheer and humor. In 1864, reviewer Ruth Hall seemed to understand Alcott's style, writing that the book's "genuine humor and pathos are nearly related." She elaborated: "'Soldiers cry for them,' (Mrs. [sic] Alcott's Hospital Sketches, I mean,) at least they would had they any idea how charming, how amusing, how sprightly they are and so pathetic withal." Hall praised Alcott's work for proceeding "without imparting the melancholy coloring" and admitted to her own physical reaction to the book, explaining that upon reading, "the facial muscles began to relax, forehead grew smoother, lips curled upward," and she started to laugh. Another reviewer wrote in 1865 that *Hospital Sketches* possessed a "sprightly humor" (*The Independent*, February 16, 1865), and yet another that the *Sketches* were "remarkable for a humor and insight which ought to have made them much more widely known" (*Harper's* January 21, 1865).[19] In addition, Alcott was very pleased to receive a letter in 1863 from Henry James Sr., father of the novelist and the philosopher, that he had enjoyed her "'charming pictures of hospital service.'" She also heard from the religious writer, David Atwood Wasson, who expressed his pleasure in the book, "written with such extraordinary wit & felicity of style" (*Journals* 123, 124).

Further, her publisher ran a large ad in *American Literary Gazette and Publishers' Circular* that contained five different testimonies, including a paragraph of praise from James, and also this sentence from *Boston Transcript*: "Fluent and sparkling in style, with touches of quiet humor and lively wit, relieving what would otherwise be a topic too somber and sad" (*American Literary Gazette* September 1, 1863). This Boston reviewer clearly understood Alcott's project of reporting through rose-colored glasses, and commented further that the *Sketches* showed "the contrast between the comic incidents and the tragic experience of a single night" (*Gazette* 1863). It would hardly have been possible to analyze Alcott's style with more accuracy—the play of the cheerfulnesses against the dismals—than if she had expressed it herself.

The Dismals

Nurse Periwinkle's singular, alacritous tone formed the initial voice of *Hospital Sketches*; but while Alcott kept the cheer at a high pitch, her tone also roiled with the less conscious voice of the "dismals." Despite Alcott's claim that the cheerfulnesses were a part of her religion she wanted "to look well after" and that the dismals were a part she wanted "to shift for themselves," the dismals nonetheless entered the narrative and, in an important way, contributed to its depth and texture.[20] Perhaps because Alcott so heartily stifled the sorrowful part of existence, the dismals appeared without her ability to foresee or manage them.[21] In the character of Trib, she failed to uphold an esprit de corps at every single moment, necessarily succumbing to depletions of energy in the form of bizarre visions and errant passions. The dismals may have had to shift for themselves, but shift they did, gaining in bleak vitality, to the point that Alcott indeed did not need to look after them at all, for they did well enough on their own. In other words, for all her playfulness, Alcott's attempt to balance and contain the unities proved in the end subject to discontinuities, the cheerfulnesses to fractures, the irrepressible views to scenes of affliction that couldn't be assuaged.

In the early travel scenes, often jocular, Tribulation also experienced an eruption of the dismals during a night voyage by rail when her imaginings emerged and turned sharply into grim fantasies. These protrusions of grimness occurred as Tribulation viewed the seemingly neutral terrain, described as "nothing to be seen outside" and "nothing inside"—nothing, that is, until she experienced a sudden eruption of perception in the form of "every variety of bunch into which the human form can be twisted, rolled, or 'massed'" (13). In this nightmarish and prescient vision Alcott marked the chaos of twisted human forms massed in sleep, forms that anticipated her later encounters with the sickness and death of the incoming wounded. During the same night, Trib experienced a second vision of mass destruction after she secured a berth on a boat, and was looking out between the draperies at the belongings of her fellow travelers: "their boots and shoes, in every imaginable attitude, assert themselves below, as if their owners had committed suicide in a body"

(14). This second image likewise intimated the dismals, the chill and anxiety that underlay Trib's otherwise bright tone. During this night of travel she surrendered more than once to morbidity, at one time thinking her "hour had come" (15). Alcott's early rosy inflections here revealed a bravado used to cover and check the fear of moving to a new location and a strange, difficult job. In these travel scenes, the dismals arose in brief moments to destabilize her rosy outlook.[22]

Any piece of American literature written during the Civil War necessarily dealt with the disturbing vision of a chaotic republic supplanting ordinary antebellum life, and Alcott dealt with such visions by describing these corporeal images during the night—the twisting human forms and the mass suicide of bodies—merging them with the nightmarish unconscious of the country. She swung between optimism and bleakness, an oscillation that defined the course of her career as a writer, too, given that she produced on the one hand novels instructive and suitable for children, and on the other hand gothic tales, macabre and grotesque. She had begun to write such gothic stories during 1863, the year of working on *Hospital Sketches*, and continued to produce "lurid thrillers" throughout the 1860s (Stern, *Journals* 20). The cheerfulnesses and the dismals located opposing emotional states that occupied the author's mind, as well as the national psyche. For Alcott, liveliness or dread predominated at any given moment to reveal her distinctive authorial voice.

She accentuated this destabilizing dichotomy by titling two abridging chapters, "A Day" and "A Night," opening the latter chapter by presenting Trib's confession that she was "fond of the night side by nature" (32), in consequence of which she was assigned the second shift. She mitigated her claim of affinity with the night by mentioning that because laughter is the best cure she had been able to sweep "the dumps and dismals" out of her ward; still she was unable to sustain her rosy view after all the coworkers had left for the night, and the ghouls and goblins, so to speak, started to come out during the after hours. Alcott recast the night patients in *Hospital Sketches* to fill the place of stock characters from gothic tales, introducing ghosts, apparitions, and phantoms.[23] Many of these characters functioned as liminal beings caught between the homefront and warfront.

One of the ghost characters was the night watchman, whom Trib "regarded with a certain awe," for she "never fairly saw" his face when he was "gliding noiselessly about the dimly lighted rooms" and "haunting the old hotel in search of its lost mates" (33). Other apparitions appeared as well: a goblin, a phantom "'all in white,'" (37), and another phantom with one leg and a "wound-fever" that left him without his wits. The one-legged phantom, "scantily draped in white," approached Trib as he "flourished a mug in one hand, an old boot in the other, calling them canteen and knapsack" (36). With this image Alcott reprised the word "knapsack," which she used in her witty conflation of homefronts and warfronts, but here his boot was a knapsack, the metaphoric parts not equaling the unities at all, but revealing a crazed confusion in which wordplay had ground down to insanity. Tribulation's earlier metaphor overlapped travel bag and knapsack to create gaiety, but this metaphor mistook a boot for a knapsack to create deep regret for the war's waste; the boot he flourished was meant to substitute for his missing, phantom leg. Though Tribulation called the night shift activities her "nocturnal adventures," the adventures failed to assuage the pain she witnessed as wounded men sleepwalked through the ward. Thus did Alcott show the nightmare side of things, apparitions rising to dispel the unities. The dismals that had been left to "shift" for themselves appeared, irrepressibly, in the form of soldier phantoms during the dark night of the war hospital.

Alcott's night scene proved preternaturally uncanny, in the sense of Freud's uncanny, as arising from those things most ordinary and homey that have returned to haunt us.[24] Trib admitted that she inhabited a "strange life" composed of sleeping "half the day, exploring Washington the other half, and all night hovering . . . over the slumbering sons of man" (34). As she surveyed the sleeping faces, many of which "became wonderfully interesting when unconscious" (34), she invoked the most haunting aspect of the uncanny, the subterranean mind returning to itself. It was as if in this setting she could glean a hidden truth of the war that magnified the underside of the nation's psyche: "some grew sad and infinitely pathetic, as if the pain borne silently all day, revenged itself by now betraying what the man's pride had concealed so well" (34–35). The masks dissolved in the dark, the suffering showed with painful clarity, and Trib "learned to know these men better by night than through any intercourse by day" (35).

Interracial Interactions

Louisa May Alcott had been raised to invest her energies in abolitionism. At home in Massachusetts she met fugitive and freed slaves, largely because of the Alcott family's extensive involvement in antislavery politics: she studied with a black schoolmate, along with her mother taught black women to read, and heard Harriet Tubman speak (Elbert, *Louisa May Alcott* xvi, x, xxvi). Alcott wrote that she "became an Abolitionist at a very early age," perhaps as a result of having been "saved from drowning in the Frog Pond . . . by a colored boy," and she had another childhood memory of "a 'contraband' hidden in the oven" of her family home (Cheney 28, 29). She wrote *Hospital Sketches* for an antislavery audience and would have considered her readers to be almost as steeped as she in the rhetoric of abolitionism. Her publisher, Redpath, obviously thought so too, as he notably advertised her work in 1863 in the abolitionist magazine *The Liberator* (along with ads in other periodicals, including *The Round Table*, *The Independent*, and *American Literary Gazette and Publishers' Circular*).

In fact, Alcott likened Tribulation Periwinkle's antislavery fervor to that of well-known abolitionist speaker Abby Folsom, stating that Trib "asserted the right of free speech as doggedly as the irrepressible Folsom herself" (59). Tribulation offered in *Hospital Sketches* an impromptu "antislavery lecture" ignited by her disdain for white nurses who were "willing to be served by the colored people, but seldom thanked them, never praised, and scarcely recognized them in the street" (58). Alcott created a flurry of a kitchen scene in which to give this speech, aimed particularly at an intolerant white nurse who was horrified when Tribulation, while stirring a pot, happened "to catch up a funny little black baby, who was toddling about the nurses' kitchen" (59). Trib delighted in this action, her enjoyment arising at least in part from her ability to rattle the white nurse, who reacted with a "sniff of disapprobation" (59).[25] In haranguing the nurse and kissing the baby, Trib delivered her own abolitionist rheto-

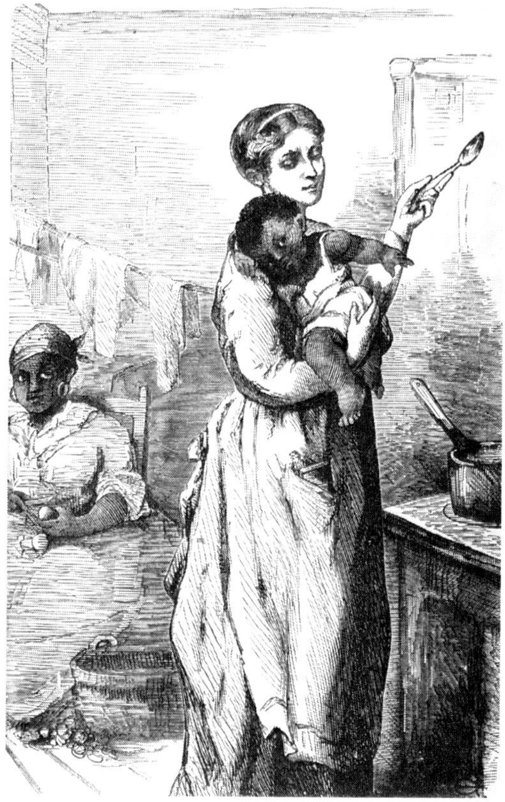

Tribulation Periwinkle and baby, captioned "One hand stirred gruel for sick America, and the other hugged baby Africa."

Louisa May Alcott, *Hospital Sketches, and Camp and Fireside Stories*, 1869

ric, extemporizing on liberation. Alcott stirred the pot, literally and figuratively, in the middle of the scene. Unfortunately, Trib's actions did not seem to edify her sniffing coworker: "This rash act, and the anti-slavery lecture that followed, while one hand stirred gruel for sick America, and the other hugged baby Africa, did not produce the cheering result which I fondly expected" (59). In fact, Trib reported, "my comrade henceforth regarded me as a dangerous fanatic" (59). This scene fixed the complexity of race discourse and race interactions in the Civil War hospital milieu.

For an example of the convoluted nature of race interactions in the 1860s hospital, we can look at the 1869 version of Alcott's 1863 book, published six years later as *Hospital Sketches, and Camp and Fireside Stories*. This later version provided a literal illustration of Nurse Periwinkle stirring the pot—a drawing that may well have undercut what Alcott wanted her readers to register about Tribulation as a committed abolitionist.[26] Perhaps because of the difficulty of focusing Alcott's complex authorial tone, the artist represented Tribulation grasping a spoon and raising it out of the baby's reach.[27] The withheld spoon formed the center of the action: an object of unfulfilled desire. Though an infant, the child knew to continue to reach for it in the sustaining belief that he deserved access to nourishment. The watchful eye of the woman in the background, probably the boy's mother, indicated that she, too, thought he deserved access, but in the illustration Tribulation was the one deciding who received resources. Elizabeth Young also interprets the scene as an unfortunate one regarding African Americans' struggle to obtain rights, noting shrewdly that the black child "functions as a figure to be civilized" (93), and that Tribulation dispenses lessons in the goal of such "civilizing."

The illustration of the two adult women, black and white, mirrored the historical reality of stratified positions for black and white nurses during the Civil War, in that the fugitive slave woman paring fruit and sitting next to the laundry performed hospital tasks often assigned to black and immigrant women. In the illustration, the oppressive implication was that the white nurse, Trib, had something to teach even the mother of the black baby about her son's care. The drawing came uncomfortably close to exemplifying the object of some of the most scathing criticisms of sentimental literature, what Michelle Burnham excoriates as "sentimental imperialism" (126): when an author or illustrator casts slave characters as minor players to accentuate the major (white) character's quandaries of sympathy about enslaved people. The illustration of Tribulation and the baby veered close to sentimental imperialism by foregrounding the white nurse, though it redeemed itself in part by showing the wonderful quickness of perception in the baby's expression.

This interpretation of the image, of course, reflected the views of the illustrator and not Alcott, though Alcott suggested in other *Hospital Sketches* scenes that she held conflicted and contradictory feelings about interracial encounters in the Civil War hospital. The scene of "baby Africa" was actually one of her most successful in depicting interracial interactions, but she represented fugitive slaves differently in other scenes, variously for background characters, for scene ambiance, and even for cheap comedy. She and many other mid-war Northern writers depicted the threshold at which black and white interactions tested abolitionist political rhetoric. Many white nurses had not met a slave or freedperson before arriving at the hospital, and some would have considered such first meetings as reckonings in which they encountered personifications of their political material, embodiments of their cause. Bruce Dorsey, for instance, points out that, "for the vast majority of white Americans in the North, slavery existed only in their imaginations" (186).

In a sense, Alcott "went to war" for the cause of abolition, the 1861 news of Sumter meaning "to Louisa and her circle less a struggle for the Union than a crusade to abolish slavery" (Jones xv). *Hospital Sketches* reflected the fact that legal changes won by and for African Americans throughout the war years were unmatched by social changes. Alcott had to modulate her responses to interracial interactions in response to quickly changing events, culminating in the Emancipation Proclamation that marked the end of her narrative. Like white many abolitionists, Alcott found herself working alongside black workers and coming face-to-face with moments of her own social intransigence, and while she fought to overcome that intransigence, she often could not override her shortcomings.

The first of such interactions occurred on her way to Washington, DC, where she described fugitive slaves as if they were players in a theatre: "We often passed colored people, looking as if they had come out of a picture book, or off the stage, but not at all the sort of people I'd been accustomed to see at the North" (17). With the phrase, "the sort of people," she implied social judgment and, further, seemed to have trouble convincing herself that the people she saw were real, a disjunction that resulted in her assigning them the role of theatrical characters. Alcott assigned black characters at times to stand in for ideas, to "function as metaphors of misrule in the service of white characters' freedoms" (Young 107). Alcott certainly described groups of black people as backdrop, what she called the "topsy-turvey" scenery, as for example when Tribulation gave her first impression of Baltimore in the dehumanizing description of the city as "full of goats, geese, colored people, and coal" (16). White abolitionists, capable of deep contradictions in behavior, "muttered racial slurs" at the same time that they espoused what might "have passed as a liberal view in the nineteenth century" (Schultz 104).

Once, in the capital city, for instance, Alcott met, in her overweening phrase, the first "genuine" African American:

> Here was the genuine article—no, not the genuine article at all, we must go to Africa for that—but the sort of creatures generations of slavery had made them: obsequious, trickish, lazy and ignorant, yet kind-hearted, merry-tempered, quick to feel and accept the least token of the brother love which is slowly teaching the white hand to grasp the black, in this great struggle for the liberty of both the races. (58)

Exhibiting a range of officious attitudes in this single description, Alcott first presumed that one human being could be more "genuine" than another; second, she employed the word "article" for a human being; and third, she used the demeaning word "creatures" (a term often used to refer to white women in the nineteenth century, too, but which rings especially distastefully here). Nonetheless, Alcott showed open-mindedness and generosity in urging equality in the last couple of lines, positing a scenario in which neither race had the upper hand and the black person could teach the white person lessons in comity. Both races interacted in harmony and "brother love," teaching "the white hand to grasp the black."

Alcott's usage of the term "article," above, reflects the opprobrious assumption built into the word "contraband," in widespread usage at the time to identify escaped slaves, and used prominently by Alcott herself in her short story "My Contraband." Existing linguistically as the legal designation for the Northern military's purported obligation to fugitive slaves, the word "contraband" functioned somewhat on the same ethical and lexical slope as the term "collateral damage" has in more recent years, both locutions relegating human beings to the status of objects of exchange in the business of war. Union General Benjamin F. Butler conceived the label early in the Civil War when pressed to make a decision concerning three fugitive slaves who had crossed the picket lines and arrived in his camp. Mostly because Butler saw those fugitives as providing free labor, he declined to return them, even though return was the legal action prescribed by the Fugitive Slave Law of 1850. Instead, he "kept the 'property,' put them to work for the Union, and sent a receipt to the owner" (Syrett 282). Soon afterward the government institutionalized the policy of legitimating the black person's change of status from "slave" to "contraband," a rewording overseen by the United States government as a way to retain, to some degree, the fugitive slave's status as property, with the overseer's privilege on the white Northern rather than the white Southern side.

The word "contraband" encrypted brutal assumptions held by many white Americans who acceded to the concept, inherent in the renaming, that fugitives were rendered objects of commercial exchange. The word ostensibly allowed Union leaders to help escapees to freedom at the same time that it benefitted the leaders by securing inexpensive labor for the war effort. Kate Masur identifies the immediate popularity of the term as a means to articulate the difficult social positioning of fugitives in Northern culture: "Most fundamentally, the new usage of 'contraband' signaled that the nation was at a crossroads. In the absence of other appropriate designations for fleeing slaves, the term was a placeholder whose appeal would fade once it became clear that the war would secure permanent emancipation" (3). Northern nurses working with fugitives in the hospitals used the vocabulary of slaveholding ownership, speaking of "their" contrabands, as Schultz points out: "It was a striking demonstration of systemic racism that women who believed slavery was a moral evil could so easily absorb its linguistic resonances" (103).

Relatively recently, contemporary sociologist Ruth Frankenberg has argued that "race shapes white women's lives" (White 1), and every person in the United States exists as part of a social system cued by racial interactions, so that no one exists apart from racial reference. Being white is hardly a neutral category but on the contrary is a position based on the coteries of privilege, the more inimical for its pretension of neutrality. Frankenberg offers three principles concerning how race shapes lives by concentrating on the unfair privilege of whiteness: the white person occupies, first of all, "a location of structural advantage, of race privilege," and second, "a 'standpoint,' a place from which white people look at ourselves, at others, and at society" (White 1).[28] These first two principles identify the location and viewpoint of race privilege, the unjust leverage whereby the white person wrongly adopts a perspective that allows her to imagine herself as neutral. Alcott and other nurses often proceeded from such a position of imagined racial neutrality, operating on unexamined assumptions of whiteness.

Alcott may have been partially aware that race patterns identity. Her first mention of meeting a black coworker in the hospital came in a flash sketch of Tribulation attempting to make her way on the hospital staircase but running into other workers such as surgeons and small boys, then becoming "hopelessly entangled in a knot of colored sisters coming to wash" (22). In this brief pass she wielded a point of view assuming white license in that she portrayed the women as a kind of scenery, linking them with the chaotic nature of hospital life, existing to define the workplace of the white nurse.[29] The meeting between Trib and the "colored sisters," however, also hinted that she felt "hopelessly entangled" in racial identity, and that in coming face-to-face and body-to-body with the women, she became aware, at least in passing, of her active involvement in such identity.

Alcott lived within daily cultural shifts that transformed personal preconceptions and as a result recorded extremely uneven responses in hospital encounters. Even as she depicted meetings as incidents that reflected the topsy-turvy hospital setting, she also reported meetings that registered positive social change. For instance, when a six-year-old black boy greeted Trib on her first day and apprised her of the goings-on in the hospital, Alcott suggested that this boy's actions were both a piece of the carnivalesque hospital setting and a reflection of the degree to which Trib's social position was in flux. Alcott also played descriptions for easy laughs, as when later she described a ten-year-old black boy sitting in a Speaker's chair of the United States Senate as the symbol par excellence for the seeming abandonment of the Capitol. Nurse Periwinkle felt yet another welter of conflicting racial outlooks as she walked through Washington, DC and surveyed the scene:

> I had not been there a week, before the neglected, devil-may-care expression in many of the faces about me seemed an urgent appeal to leave nursing white bodies, and take some care for these black souls.

> Much as the lazy boys and saucy girls tormented me, I liked them, and found that any show of interest or friendliness brought out the better traits which live in the most degraded and forsaken of us all. (58)

Stereotyping "black souls" as lazy, saucy, and tormenting, Tribulation seemed proud to act with seeming forbearance even as she spoke in stereotypes; further, when she added, "I liked them," she exhibited self-congratulation for upholding principles of seeming benevolence in understanding fugitives as "degraded and forsaken," and suggested that she as a white charity worker could garner self-esteem through such a philanthropic approach.

She was less biased, however, when positioning herself in the more abstract realm of abolitionist discourse, a realm without the complexities of personal interactions. Celebrating her antislavery heritage in direct appeal, Alcott stood up for the cause and rose to the occasion, as for instance when she asserted that, "the blood of two generations of abolitionists waxed hot in my veins, and, at the first opportunity, proclaimed itself, and asserted the right of free speech" (59). Probably the word "proclaimed" was no accident, given the anticipation of Lincoln's hallowed Proclamation. Alcott celebrated the Emancipation Proclamation of January 1, 1863, with exhilaration, memorializing what was the most momentous New Year's Eve of the era. On that night the number of fugitive slaves who had fled North to make temporary homes in Union hospitals and camps were summarily declared free. Listening to the bells ringing at midnight, Tribulation acknowledged, "I waited for New Year's day with more eagerness than I had ever known before; and, though it brought me no gift, I felt rich in the act of justice so tardily performed toward some of those about me" (59). She listened to the bells, "electrified her room-mate by dancing out of bed, throwing up the window, and flapping my handkerchief, with a feeble cheer, in answer to the shout of a group of colored men in the street below" (59).[30] Alcott (if not necessarily the men in the street) would have thought of them all as forming a group, rejoicing together, and allied by dint of her own political activities.[31] Trib recalled the evening:

> The sky was clear, the moon shone benignly, a mild wind blew across the river, and all good omens seemed to usher in the dawn of the day whose noontide cannot now be long in coming. If the colored people had taken hands and danced around the White House, with a few cheers for the much abused gentleman who has immortalized himself by one just act, no President could have had a finer levee, or one to be prouder of. (59)

Alcott pulled out all the stops, delivering auspicious signs of clear sky, bright moon, mild wind, ushered-in dawn, and coming noontide. She attempted to bolster the marred reputation of the president with a fantasy of a circle of newly freed people dancing around the White House to make of it a fine "levee," or reception. The word "levee" also derives from a French root, indicating "elevation" or "arising," so that the image of an elevated president in the middle of a people rising to freedom offered a kind of finale for *Hospital Sketches* (with only one page remaining before the postscript).

Throughout the narrative Alcott borrowed uneasily from an abolitionist discourse that reflected, often inaccurately, her encounters with individuals, as when Trib characterized herself self-deceptively as "treating the blacks as I did the whites" (58). She mixed this self-deception with resurgent idealism, as in the triumphant scene above. Though the 1863 Emancipation Proclamation was celebrated with great optimism and seemed to signal a world of possibilities, it took more than a century for African Americans to see the fruition of even the most basic rights and freedoms. In less than two years, from the start of the Civil War in April 1861 to the Proclamation in January 1863, the country underwent profound racial changes, African Americans' legal status altering from enslaved person to (in some cases) "contraband" to freedperson. The last of these developments occurred during that small time frame in the couple months that *Hospital Sketches* covered, December 1862 through January 1863, when Alcott attempted to realign her politics of abolitionism to social equality, with a new call for action based on the rights of all people.

Trib reported in the *Sketches* that she felt a desire to stop nursing white bodies "and take some care for these black souls" (58), which Alcott in fact did try to do, petitioning Thomas Wentworth Higginson in November 1863, after she returned home. She asked for his help in finding her a position to "go South & help the blacks," because it seemed to her "the greater work" (*Letters* 96). She wanted to care for freedpeople but instead, during her illness and while sequestered in her room at the Union Hotel Hospital, she was herself cared for by a black nurse: "Black women, seldom recognized as nurses, cared for sick white nurses, as Matilda Cleaver John did when Hannah Ropes and Louisa May Alcott contracted typhoid fever at Union Hotel in 1862" (Schultz 118). After leaving the hospital Alcott never engaged in the work of nursing black Americans, ultimately returning to and remaining at home in Concord.

In the few months after she returned from service, while still fighting off typhoid and the mercury used to treat it, Louisa May Alcott committed her hospital experiences to paper, writing furiously but carefully, to ensure "no offence could be took." She crafted a locution that would finally hold together the multifaceted purposes of genres and consolidate a work that would be consumed and enjoyed by many readers. Succinctly stated, there was no genre of American nurse narrative for Alcott to emulate because it hadn't yet been invented, so she found her way by timbre alone, speaking in a funny, brassy diction. One of the crucial narratological considerations of *Sketches* is how Alcott defined the literary terrain of a fictional narrator living in a nonfiction world so that she could speak her way through the chaos.

She made use of the women's rights rhetoric of her era to develop a conversation with her audience and strengthen the writer–reader bond, a bond that she reinforced by depicting scenes of motivation and travel, and showing the link between homefront and warfront. She made use of abolitionist discourse in both uneasy and somewhat successful ways, offering a complicated presentation of the state of interracial interactions in the hospital. Alcott constructed a book that "was received with universal favor," as *The Commonwealth* reported in Boston (*American Literary Gazette* September 1, 1863). In *Hospital Sketches*, Alcott created a main character, Tribulation, who experienced unexpected events that she met with humor as well as a chipper voice that pretended not to be, but was, shaken by uncertainty. With seemingly ineluctable cheer she interacted with her readers from within a tension of oscillating awareness, willing herself to overlook the dismals that would shift for themselves, even though they dragged right along with her and gave resonance to her singular voice.

Think what this would have have [sic] been, and you are ready to appreciate the relief and comfort that was. (5)

CHAPTER TWO

Georgeanna Woolsey's *Three Weeks at Gettysburg*

Connecting Links

Georgeanna Woolsey's family hoped that she, at twenty-eight years of age, would be too young to be accepted for nursing service, but Georgy, as they called her, was admitted because she left "a blank inadvertently" where she was supposed to record her age (quoted in Austin 39). The Woolseys, well-to-do and socially conscious, had taken on the work of abolition as a family commitment, and when the Civil War started they took on Union wartime work with equal fervor; Woolsey's brother, Charley, served in the army, and all seven Woolsey sisters eventually dedicated themselves to Civil War nursing. Three of them, Abby, Jane, and Georgeanna, along with two other nurses, "would go on to lead the postwar movement to establish training schools for female nurses" (Clinton and Silber 112), and are credited with inaugurating the American nursing profession. When it came her turn to serve, Georgy entered what was in effect the family business of active benevolence;[1] she stated in brisk narration the nature of her on-the-go circumstances and made clear that the motivation for her and her traveling companion was "to do what we could" (3).[2]

Georgeanna Woolsey wrote *Three Weeks at Gettysburg* with a deft hand, welcoming a caring readership to her narrative. She mentioned to her audience the travails of a trip from Baltimore to Gettysburg that took twenty-four hours instead of the usual four, and reported on "the rail-road bridge broken up by the enemy" (4). Because of the damaged bridge, soldiers who needed transportation to points beyond the Gettysburg battlefield had to endure long waits. Setting up a station to mitigate these uncomfortable circumstances, Woolsey and other workers operated a temporary lodge and kitchen to restore comfort and health to the soldiers whose access to travel was blocked. The relief workers' chief task was to establish a relief station from which the soldiers could eventually continue on their way despite the break in connections.

From the outset of her narrative, Woolsey created a conversation with her readers that depended on the image of the broken bridge and the relief station built by the United States Sanitary Commission. The link of the bridge offered a useful figure for Woolsey to narrate the nurse's service during the war, and to capture the attention of her readers she structured her narrative accordingly. At the time the commission arrived on the Gettysburg field, many more wounded men required attention than could be cared for, so surgeons had told any patients who were ambulatory to make their own way to the railroad cars, a trek of a day or two, to find other care; a number of men chose to walk to the rails to avoid the overcrowded and improvised facilities already attending to the wounded. Woolsey's conversational rhetoric prompted her readers to imagine the experience of the soldiers who faced the very real possibility of falling by the wayside, and to imagine them reaching their destination only to find the railroad cars too full, or already departed: "For the first few days the worst cases only, came down in ambulances from the hospitals; hundreds of fellows hobbled along as best they could in heat and dust, for hours, slowly toiling, and many hired farmers' wagons, as hard as the farmers' fists themselves, and were jolted down to the railroad, at

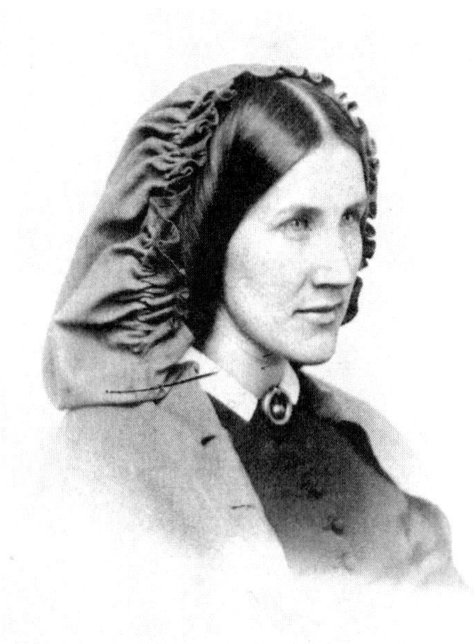

Georgeanna Woolsey

MOLLUS Massachusetts Civil War photographs, United States Army Heritage and Education Center, Carlisle, PA

three or four dollars the man" (5). Woolsey galvanized the sympathetic responses of her audience by prompting them to respond: "Think what this *would* have have [*sic*] been, and you are ready to appreciate the relief and comfort that *was*. No men were turned back" (5). She drew on the imaginations of her readership directly to pull them into an implied dialogue that she would carry on throughout.

The Sanitary Commission adopted a rescue strategy that yoked "the hospital at one end, the railroad at the other," and made "a connecting link between these two ends" (5). By easing the hardships of the exhausted and sick soldiers' journey, the commission made itself indispensible, stepping up to provide a service the government had either overlooked or been unable to supply. Woolsey took pains to articulate this scene as a powerful spur to readers to make donations to the commission's cause, reminding them that their charity underwrote the vital linkage between homefront and warfront. With the goal of channeling important resources from one front to the other, she shaped her narrative to emphasize the commonality between writer and reader. As the narrative progressed, moreover, she represented other linkages, such as those bridging people of different regions and races. In reporting the success of distributing provisions to soldiers at the bridge station, she also introduced many other kinds of connections to augment a crucial vision of relief for the nation as a whole.

The Sanitary Commission organizers prided themselves on their efficiency in arriving where they were most needed, and Woolsey acknowledged the precipitate service of women in the commission by deploying abolitionist and women's-rights rhetoric. She used the specific tactics of indirection and deflection to assert women's organizational role: "I cannot pretend to tell you what was done by all the big wheels of the concern, but only how two of the smallest ones went round, and what turned up in the going" (3). Her claim that she and her companion nurse (her mother) were small wheels may have sounded modest but served, in fact, as no small claim, given that the turn of phrase operated on a couple of registers. The "wheel" comment may well have harkened to a statement made by President Lincoln in 1861, on the occasion of agreeing to medical consultation between the government and the Sanitary Commission, whereby he agreed to allow the commission to operate during the war, albeit reluctantly, because he feared it would become "the fifth wheel on the coach" (quoted in Chambers and Anderson 634). Despite Lincoln's misgivings, the Sanitary Commission became not a fifth wheel but instead the emblem of resourcefulness and competence and a credit to Union operations.

The small wheels did big labor for the enterprise. The United States Sanitary Commission and the United States Christian Commission, the two major Civil War relief organizations, delivered and distributed to soldiers supplies that would not have been immediately available otherwise. To glean an idea of the level of the country's unpreparedness in caring for the wounded, consider that the United States had no standing army at the beginning of the Civil War and no infrastructure or sophisticated organization to support patients. There was only one full-fledged U.S. military hospital: "Before 1860, the U.S. Army had infirmaries at army posts, but only one was considered a hospital, a 40-bed unit at the military post at Fort Leavenworth in Kansas" (Dammann, Bollet 112). Under the aegis of the Sanitary Commission, an organization considered the precursor to the Red Cross, Woolsey and other workers provided food, clothing, medicine, bandages, and bedding to soldiers. Implying that the United States could not yet come to the rescue as nimbly as the commission, Woolsey asserted that her group arrived "as usual, just where the Government had left off" (4). Women nurses by and large lavished praise on the Sanitary Commission, including Anna Morris Holstein, also at Gettysburg, who claimed that the organization was "ever ready and anxious to fill up all demands which the government *could not*" (Holstein 41). Woolsey focused on the small wheels of the operation, using the figure of the "smallest" wheels to emphasize that women nurses were an integral part of an in-motion machine that contributed vitally to the whole. She accentuated the fact that the commission depended on those workers of seemingly minimal importance—the female movers who performed essential relief work. Woolsey was but one of many thousands vitally concerned with keeping a steady influx of provisions arriving, and she kept them coming by appealing to women readers and prompting their involvement in the large project of the commission.

Woolsey was altogether aware of the power of rhetoric; in a letter she wrote the month after the battle at Gettysburg she explained that she was urged to write *Three Weeks*, explicitly "meant to 'fire the hearts' of the sewing circles, which all over the country, were keeping up the Sanitary Commission supplies" (Woolsey, Hoisington 316). Available in the late summer of 1863 (after Alcott's pieces in *The Commonwealth*, but a few weeks before the book, *Hospital Sketches*), Woolsey's brief but vibrant twenty-four page *Three Weeks at Gettysburg* was printed and reprinted for the purpose of soliciting donations. On its title page she stated forthrightly the narrative's intended audience: "This unpretending sketch of the labors of two Ladies among the wounded, after the Battle of Gettysburg, was originally printed for private distribution among a few of the Soldiers' Aid Societies." Woolsey also explained on the title page that the narrative had now been reproduced for "a more general circulation" among friends and United States Sanitary Commission contributors.

The anonymous document was circulated among the local chapters of aid societies, and the commission ordered "10,000 copies for distribution" (Woolsey, Hoisington 316).

Despite being nearly defunct within its first year of operations, the USSC found that it could boost donations by soliciting heavily after major battles, when the public was on high alert. The Union citizenry, for instance, demanded news in particular of Gettysburg, the battle that frightened and convinced Northerners that their homeland was not secure from Confederate invasion. Garnering a response in *The North American Review*, Woolsey's *Three Weeks* was described by a critic as a work that could "be read in a few minutes, but will compare in interest with anything which has been written about the battle" ("Critical" 266). The narrative was passed around, Katharine Wormeley including it entire in her own 1863 *The United States Sanitary Commission*, asserting that the embedded narrative was "written by the woman best fitted for the work, and best fitted to tell of it" (Wormeley 123). Savvy in promoting Woolsey's work, the Sanitary Commission announced the narrative's availability in the *Saturday Evening Post*, and explained that they would "forward copies of these publications [including *Three Weeks*] to any persons desiring them who will send their address" (November 7, 1863). The narrative was free on written request. Giesberg asserts that *The Sanitary Commission Bulletin* "enjoyed a generous circulation and a wide, largely female readership," adding that "one local woman noted that a popular commission publication written by Georgeanna Woolsey . . . was returned to her 'at the end of the month . . . literally worn out'" (*Sisterhood* 104).

Woolsey's frequent lists of items of provisions showed her frank acknowledgement of the commission's boosterism and attention to readers' contributions. She chronicled the distribution of a surplus of items to soldiers, such as "socks, slippers, shirts, drawers" (11), and also crutches, pads, soap, towels, drinks, and food. In one instance, she elaborated on the pleasant stir created when soldiers received a shipment of "coveted dressing gowns" (11): "Such pride they felt in them! comparing colors, and smiling all over as they lay in clean and comfortable rows ready for supper, 'on dress parade,' they used to say" (11). The dispensing of cologne also produced a desired commotion, the scent going "right to the

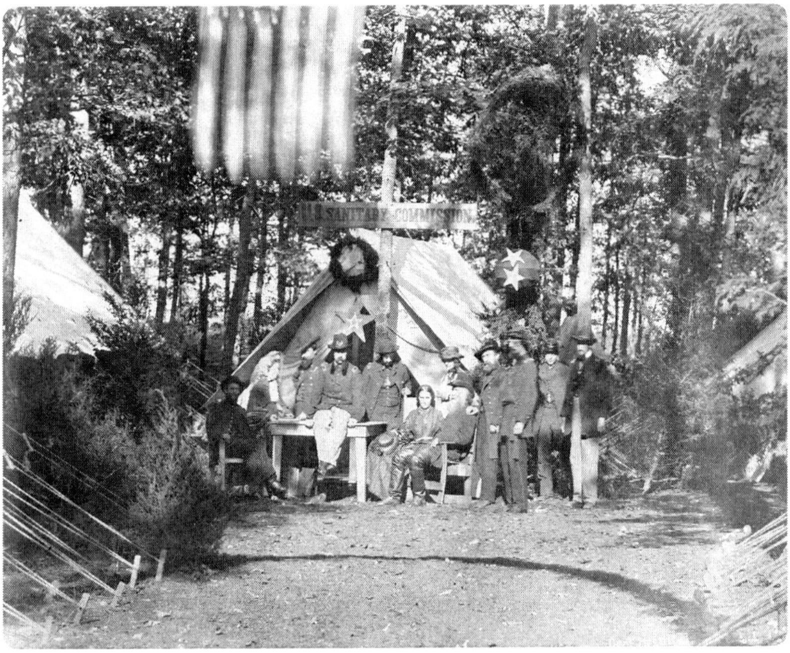

Sanitary Commission at Gettysburg General Hospital, 1863

Courtesy of the Library of Congress

noses and hearts of the men" (11). In yet another list, Woolsey inventoried sweet foods: "jelly-pots and bottles of all kinds of good syrups, blackberry and black currant." Most crucially, she spoke to those readers who might continue to provide needed materials: "Barrels were ranged round the tent walls; shirts, drawers, dressing-gowns, socks, and slippers (I wish we had more of the latter), rags and bandages . . . boxes of tea, coffee, soft crackers, tamarinds, cherry brandy, etc." As straightforwardly as possible, she talked slippers to her readers.

The compendiums of provisions indicate how successfully Woolsey joined the energies of those at the homefront and the warfront to bridge audience and soldier for the larger cause of war relief. In place of the broken bridge that could not convey the soldiers to safety or home, Woolsey, with the help of her readers, constructed a bridge of aid that provided a few comforts of home in the interim. Her purpose consisted in depicting a linking structure for her readers, but being the abolitionist she was, she took on another purpose as well, which was to evoke a bridge between peoples of the nation. Woolsey's narrative espoused linkage not only between homefront and warfront but between blacks and whites and between Northerners and Southerners. Despite the fact that these linkages were not always categorically easy for her audience to imagine, Woolsey invited the attempt. The act of reading about others' circumstances allowed the nineteenth-century reader imaginative activity, in that "the world of print may in fact have been one of the few places where people of different classes and culture could encounter one another across boundaries, boundaries of the imagination if no other" (Sicherman, "Reading" 151). Woolsey attempted to cross such boundaries by documenting interracial and inter-regional encounters. Having established a conversation with her readers, she fortified that bond and used it to connect other groups.

WOOLSEY WAS GIVEN ample opportunities at the Gettysburg site to attempt the bridging of races, having met a number of freedpeople employed by the Sanitary Commission as laborers. Some of these meetings revealed that her abolitionist work did not exempt her from personal limitations in tolerance, similarly to Alcott, who exhibited actions that tested and belied her abolitionist roots. Also like Alcott, Woolsey wrote and published her 1863 narrative in the year Lincoln signed the Emancipation Proclamation, an act that both regenerated and complicated white abolitionists' sense of purpose, prompting them to revise their efforts from militating for an end to slavery to pressing for economic and social justice. Advocating for social justice did not happen automatically, and most reformists struggled to reconceive their political work, as "they began to grapple more substantially with the question of what place freed slaves were going to fill after the war and emancipation" (Sizer 147). After the war they would reframe rhetoric in terms of political and economic advancement and begin to mobilize for social changes to keep in step with legal changes, but during the war decade, the activism and the discourse were in flux.

Woolsey wrestled tacitly with these questions, as in this portrayal of black laborers preparing food for the soldiers at the commission's railroad camp:

> Here we set up two stoves, with four large boilers, always kept full of soup and coffee, watched by four or five black men, who did the cooking, under our direction, and sang (not under our direction) at the tops of their voices all day. (6)

By using generalizations to describe their activities (they "always" kept the food at the ready, and sang "at the tops" of their voices, and cooked and sang "all day"), Woolsey employed diction that threatened to capture the newly emancipated men in something like mythological stasis. Woolsey appeared to test her ability to place her own female agency against the black men's agency, stating that they did the cooking "under our direction," while they sang "(not under our direction)" (6). With the parenthetical stab at humor, she gestured toward workplace power differences in the unsettled way Alcott did. Margaret Creighton interprets Woolsey's sentence as indicating power leveraging in which white workers note black compliance, "—or they thought it was compliance" (153). In attempting to assign interracial positioning as either "under our direction" or "(not under our direction)," one of Woolsey's concerns appeared to be who supervised whom.

Despite keeping track of direction, she more or less honored their singing, offering a sampling of two songs newly popular during the war: "Oh darkies hab you seen my Massa," and "When this *cruel* war is *over*" (6–7). Both songs, written in 1862, addressed issues of black liberation, overtly in the case of the first (actually named "Kingdom Coming," written by Henry Clay Work), which "celebrated the advent of emancipation" (Miller 172). The second song, "When This Cruel War Is Over," written by Charles C. Sawyer, was "the most popular song of the Civil War," selling "over one million copies of sheet music" (Manning 213). Sung by both Union and Confederate soldiers, the plaintive melody was recast with minor changes in lyrics to suit blue or gray uniform color. Woolsey reported the title line with the words "*cruel*" and "*over*" italicized, perhaps to show the singers' emphatic delivery, but the men may instead have weighted the words to suggest their own point of view. Accentuating these lyrics, the newly emancipated freedpeople may have sung about lives long involved in a cruel war against slavery—a war in which they were still in actuality involved, despite the Proclamation. Such irony is commensurate with the "Signifyin(g)" Henry Louis Gates Jr. identifies as the black hero's "sign of the triumph of wit and reason, his language of Signifyin(g) standing as the linguistic sign of the ultimate triumph of self-consciously formal language use" (77).

In an even more racially complex scene, Woolsey described a group of freedmen working in a field in which she and others had just buried a soldier: "a number of colored freedmen, working for Government, on the railroad, had their camp, and every night they took their recreation after the heavy work of the day was over, in prayer meetings. Such an 'inferior race,' you know!" (18). Motioning to her readers that as a fervent antislavery proponent she gave unequivocal support to the freedmen, the born-and-raised abolitionist Woolsey no doubt felt immense gratification that she and her audience could affirm mutual disapprobation of damaging racial stereotypes. She telegraphed this rapport with her audience in the bantering phrase, "you know!" On the other hand, though, she agreed with Harriet Beecher Stowe in seeing religious devotion as a primary racial characteristic of Africans; Stowe told her readers that of "'all races of the earth, none have received the Gospel with such eager docility,'" and Riss observes that her understanding of the black reception of religion "very carefully defines this distinctive feature as biological" (64). Stowe was misguided in attributing genetic reasons to religious devotion, when a number of reasons, including political, could have attracted enslaved people to the message of liberty embedded in some forms of Christian expression. For example, hymns and interpretations of scriptural passages offered a means of political action through black Signifying that promoted a veiled resistance.

One night Woolsey and other white workers attended such a Christian service in the tent of freedpeople who sang and prayed "with all their souls, as only black men and slaves can: for themselves and for the dear, white people who had come over to the meeting, and for 'Massa Lincoln,' for whom they seemed to have a reverential affection, some of them a sort of worship, which confused Father Abraham and Massa Abraham . . ." (19). Whereas many former bondspeople expressed veneration for Lincoln because he delivered the Emancipation Proclamation, those at the church meeting were unlikely to have conflated the U. S. Abraham Lincoln with the Biblical father figure Abraham, given that the Biblical figure was distinguished by having left his native land to live in a strange country, just as enslaved people had been thrust from theirs. They might have chosen, however, to connect the two father figures for good political purpose, one Abraham emancipating slaves, and the other building a home in a new land as Africans had been forced to do. Woolsey seemed predisposed to understand black culture as one of simplicity rather than of rich insight and irony.

In Gettysburg, some of the black population were newly freed slaves, but many were longtime residents of Pennsylvania, as Creighton shows in her detailed study of Gettysburg during the war. Arguing convincingly that there existed "multiple dimensions of black civilian experience during the Gettysburg episode of the Civil War" (135), Creighton demonstrates that members of the black community had settled in the area, including workers such as farm owners, shop clerks, hotel workers, cooks, and others. Many of these townspeople went into hiding until the conflict was over, while others succeeded in evacuating before the battle, out of fear of being recaptured by Rebel soldiers. Creighton confirms that after the Battle of Gettysburg, "black men, some local and some employed from outside the borough, helped rebuild the railroads" (152), but many were not necessarily manual laborers before the war. This complex picture of the black residents at Gettysburg resituates perceptions of those who worked at the battle site: some were undoubtedly recently former slaves, but many were Pennsylvania residents with standing in their community.

Mindful of these multiple social dimensions, we can interpret one of Woolsey's stories that seems meant to be about the kindness of white nurses but may show the nurses' attempt at racial and social placement that can accompany benevolence activities. In an activity instigated and undertaken by women relief workers who saw the black workers as being "grateful for every little thing," one of the women bought and hemmed "several dozen bright handkerchiefs" (19). They were set out on the table after a prayer meeting, and the freedmen approached, one by one, to choose a kerchief. Each of them, wrote Woolsey, coveted the one yellow kerchief among the purple and blue ones, prizing it for its "particular pumpkin color." She asserted that the freedmen, after choosing their handkerchiefs, tied them on their heads and sang a last song, "keeping time, all round, with blue and purple and yellow nods" (20). The uncomfortable assumptions in this story are compounded when we remember that not all freedmen came from the same background and hence not all were motivated by the same desires in selecting and wearing kerchiefs; some may have been established Gettysburg townspeople with longstanding Pennsylvania residence and businesses of their own, while some may have been newly enfranchised men who had escaped from a Southern state; the simple gift of a kerchief would have meant something radically different to those of divergent social backgrounds. It is also possible that the scene of keeping time and nodding evidenced a sophisticated incident of Signifying. Much as Woolsey attempted to use narrative strategies that demonstrated linkage between black and white people, the attempts were often, as in this case, displays of advantage —the whiteness Frankenberg describes as a perspective of seeming neutrality, which actually reveals privilege.

REGARDING LINKAGE in relations between North and South, Woolsey attended both Union and Confederate patients and clearly fostered the idea that proximity in the hospital could prompt closer association or, as she put it, each could become "better friends" with the other. While it was not unusual in Civil War literature to convey the occasional concord between Union and Confederate men, the sentiment was more widely propounded after the war than during it. In her narrative Woolsey generated a particularly early instance of how a coalescing national identity could be forged through the terms of conflict. She tried to be fair to Northern and Southern patients alike, a policy the United States Sanitary Commission, which expected its workers to show impartiality, encouraged. Charles Janeway Stillé stated in the somewhat self-congratulatory

1866 bulletin that summarized the commission's work during the war: "Everything that human kindness could devise was gathered up by the wide benevolence of this Commission, and poured out among the wounded soldiers, friend and foe alike" (*The United States Sanitary Commission* 43). Woolsey also suggested in her own reporting that soldiers interacted harmoniously, fraternally even, in their common ground of suffering.

After the carnage on the field at Gettysburg, wounded survivors lay alongside one another in the hospitals, both Northerners and Southerners together under the nurses' care. The Southerners spoke in gentlemanly tones and Woolsey responded in kind:

> "Have you friends in the army, madam?" a rebel soldier, lying on the floor of the car, said to me, as I gave him some milk. "Yes, my brother is on ——'s staff." "I thought so, ma'am. You can always tell; when people are good to soldiers they are sure to have friends in the army." (9–10)

The maternal nurse provided milk to the gracious enemy soldier while he spoke of the compassion instilled by the existence of family. In other scenarios, soldiers expressed surprise at Woolsey's kindness, one saying, "We are rebels, you know, ma'am," and another, "Do you treat rebels so?" Here, the Confederate soldier was taken aback by the Northern stance of fairness, intimating that he believed Southern women would have been less forgiving if the roles were reversed. Woolsey played on the benevolent Christian sympathies of her Northern readers at the same time that she valorized the perception of Northern nurses' acts of impartiality. In Woolsey's sanguine model of the United States, camaraderie and nurturance operated in the midst of disorder:

> It was strange to see the good brotherly feeling come over the soldiers, our own and the rebels, when side by side they lay in our tents. "Hullo, boys! this is the pleasantest way to meet, isn't it? We are better friends when we are as close as this, than a little farther off." (10)

Woolsey reasoned that propinquity necessitated close interactions, that humankind need only become acquainted, share milk perhaps, in order to find amity.

Woolsey also foregrounded a moment of local civilian discord to accentuate soldier unity, offering the vignette of a local Gettysburg man of Dutch descent, whom she contrasted to the harmonious military men. The local man, who "came creeping" into the camp because he "'had never seen a rebel'" (13) was portrayed by Woolsey to be ignorant and craven because he was unable to see Southerners as human beings. She contrasted this civilian's behavior with the bravery of the Rebel soldiers in the hospital tent. The man's cowardice was exposed by a woman, who asked him provocatively why he hadn't seen a rebel before, why he hadn't taken his "'gun and helped to drive them out of [his] town?'" (13). At the woman's comment, the Confederate soldiers roared with laughter, the entire camp joining in to disparage the man's behavior. The tale ended with a brace of warmth among Union and Confederate soldiers reacting together, the moral of the tale proved not by invective but laughter.

The most trenchant scene of Northern and Southern harmony occurred during the late-afternoon arrival of more than 100 wounded Confederate soldiers, to whom Woolsey and her coworkers ministered throughout the night. One of these patients in particular was failing, and Woolsey took interest in him, equating the Southern man with a Northern soldier because of his beauty: "a fair-haired, blue-eyed young lieutenant, a face innocent enough for one of our own New England boys" (16). She wrote that her impartial view of the man arose from the fact that "I could not think of him as a rebel, he was too near heaven for that" (16). Many critics have analyzed Louisa May Alcott's attention to one of her patients, John, whom she helped to experience the nineteenth-century "good death" that functioned as the fruition of a person's life; Faust characterizes the "Good Death" as modeling Jesus and "giving up one's soul" with gladness (6).[3] The ability to ease a soldier's final time so as to find peace in his last minutes formed a major narrative convention in several nurse narratives. Woolsey demonstrated to her readers that the female nurse was remarkable for helping the common soldier—including the Confederate soldier—experience a meaningful death.

In Woolsey's story, the soldier had been unable to eat for days, and the young man asked for nothing, but Woolsey was able to prompt him to take nourishment: "I coaxed him to try a little milk gruel, made nicely with lemon and brandy, and one of the satisfactions of our three weeks is the remembrance of the empty cup I took away afterward, and his perfect enjoyment of that supper" (16). In a maternal and almost luminous gesture she offered the enemy a final meal, for which the soldier thanked her profusely, talking for hours into the night about his "'good supper'" (16). This poignant exchange between friend and foe, Northern nurse and Southern soldier, revealed a shared connection of Christian values and maternal generosity. Woolsey took pains to employ redemptive iconography for the nurses' work that benefited not only their own men, but the "enemy." She reported that the man spoke "in a pleased, childlike way," until midnight, when "the change came . . . and in the morning they found him "sliding out of our care" (16–17).

During the war death was often sudden, anonymous, disordered, and without consolation; indeed, as Faust points out, "Civil War battlefields and hospitals could have provided the material for an exemplary text on how not to die" (9). But Woolsey's story showcased an unusually good death, in which she, representing a gesture of supernal generosity, helped a Confederate soldier find meaningful passage. As the man slipped into his last hours he retraced his childhood, recounted battles, and sang wordless songs, but the scene at this point took an unlikely turn. During his decline he was recognized, and his brother was found and brought to witness so that, by fortuitous coincidence, the man experienced a death replete with an actual family member present. Woolsey described the scene with the added narrative touch that his death occurred at sunset: "The Lord *had* mercy, and at sunset I put my hand on the lieutenant's heart, to find it still" (18). Many Union nurse narratives retrieved an iconic scene of redemption from among many instances of carnage, describing a Union soldier's good death taking place under the aegis of the woman relief worker; Woolsey's *Three Weeks* brought this solace to a Confederate soldier, in a profound attempt to portray and advocate for regional linkage to her readers.

Woolsey created different cultural bridges in *Three Weeks*, including her attempts to link black and white, North and South, homefront and warfront. We will now circle back to this last link, for while we have observed how the homefront came to the warfront when civilians provided donations, we have not seen the obverse—how the warfront came to the homefront. In a powerful example of conversational discourse, Woolsey offered to her audience an anecdote of the domestic line holding firm in the face of encroaching gunfire. This anecdote portrayed a Gettysburg girl who was caught in the middle of an attack yet stayed steadfastly at her domestic work, despite the danger. Described as "a red-cheeked, strong, country girl," the young woman stood her ground when shells started to fly, as she was baking for the soldiers and the dough was rising: "I couldn't leave my bread. When the first shell came in at the window and crashed through the room, an officer came and said, 'you had better get out of this,' but I told him I *could not* leave my bread . . ." (14). When the second and third shells entered the house, she finally repaired to the cellar, but left the bread in the oven, again declaring that she didn't want to leave the house because if she did, "the rebels would a come in and daubed the dough all over the place" (14).

Woolsey applauded the girl's bravery and considered her actions the triumph of a woman under siege, as her dooryard became a battlefield. The girl's courage was underscored by the permeability of the boundaries between the domestic and military arenas. Woolsey used the grimly humorous vignette to tout the example of female conviction to her audience and to plant a model of women's rights. The story resonated with the story of Jenny Wade, a similar tale of a woman baking bread in Gettysburg, though Woolsey's narrative predated the 1864 publication of the poem, *Jenny Wade of Gettysburg*, published by Mary Eastman. Eastman's Jenny Wade differed in that Wade died from a Rebel bullet while she was baking bread, whereas Woolsey's Gettysburg girl purveyed the primacy of woman's labor in a seriocomic story of preparing the staff of life in an active war zone. Woolsey's girl lived to beat the odds, and her tale stood in for the Northern women at home who performed less heroic but equally useful feats by contributing food for the war effort. Woolsey counted on her readers to identify with the girl.

OF THE SEVEN nurse narrators studied in this project, no other so confidently acknowledged her readers as Georgeanna Woolsey, who used a familiar and straightforward second-person voice: "You fed and sheltered them just when no one else could have done so; and out of the boxes and barrels of good and nourishing things, which you people at home had supplied, we took all that was needed" (6). Woolsey bridged writer and audience by both soliciting and thanking them for donating the supplies that were of paramount importance in making the difference between life and death for soldiers. Her narrative voice appointed the recipients of her words as the givers of an implied cornucopia of goods, her sense of audience specific, her conversational rhetoric direct. Interestingly, while her sense of audience was indeed specific, her own narrative voice, robust as it was, did not divulge her identity. Woolsey's mode of addressing a designated audience remained forthright, but the claim of authorship was deflected. This combination of an extremely particular readership addressed by an effaced author resulted in the creation of an anomalous narrative field. Many nineteenth-century women, acutely aware that the choice of anonymity (or pseudonymity) could have a profound effect on the reception of their work and their readership, made such decisions in order to shape a desired response. When Katherine Wormeley included Woolsey's narrative in her own book on the USSC, she respected Woolsey's decision to remain anonymous and declined to divulge her identity.

While anonymity might be viewed as a position of weakness or a retreat from claiming one's own literary product, it is also a strategy by which an author claims power by presenting her work as she wishes it to be received. Alexis Easley asserts that a woman bypassing authorial recognition can "both construct and subvert notions of individual authorial identity, manipulating the publishing conventions associated with various print media for personal and professional advantage" (2). It seems plausible that Woolsey adopted anonymity for *Three Weeks at Gettysburg* because she wanted to purvey a stance of selflessness befitting her culture's conceptions of the ideal, modest female, the screen of anonymous, unassuming supplicant a useful promotional tactic to attract and stimulate fundraising. A writer–reader bond based on authorial absence offered the possibility of an unusual textual collaboration into which the reader could lean imaginatively, and contribute generously. A woman writer could use anonymity, as Woolsey did, to negotiate from a modest platform and espouse a particular civic cause.

She chose not to divulge her name, but it soon came to light. The shift of *Three Weeks at Gettysburg* from anonymity to a dawning recognition of Woolsey's identity, in fact, caused something of a stir among her family members. Caroline Woolsey ribbed her sister about the popularity of the work: "Door-bell—Miss E. M. wants to know if I wrote those everlasting *Three Weeks at Gettysburg*. . . . We think of opening a branch office of information and drawing a salary from the Sanitary Commission . . . What it is to be the sister of an authoress!" (Hoisington 597). Georgeanna Woolsey had tried but not succeeded in remaining nameless, and it could have been that her family's prestige was too difficult to conceal for long. Behind the screen of namelessness, Woolsey had been able to implore and congratulate a specific audience in clear, warm, familiar prose, and they had responded. The fact of anonymity set up a singular dynamic in which the writer was ambiguous and the reader was unequivocally spurred to motivation. That dynamic, while it lasted, produced active response.

Woolsey bolstered the conversational bond between writer and reader further by using a hint of the epistolary form at the narrative's outset. As if she were posting a letter to a recipient, she adopted the formulation, "Dear ———" (3). The technique of writing an open-ended letter was a frequent literary technique used in nineteenth-century texts but, given its ability to instill familiarity, to employ it in a fundraising narrative further nudged and invited the audience. Woolsey used the powerful second-person voice several times to specify, both directly and indirectly, the commission's need for donations. The epistolary convention conveyed intimacy, creating a kind of write-in inducement for the donor to imagine herself inscribed in the text.

Not only did Woolsey mold an unassuming authorial identity by declining to identify herself, she also fashioned a unique first-person plural address, a kind of double anonymity, using "we" to include the other woman she worked with, also unnamed, both mentioned as the "two ladies" on the title page. Woolsey withheld the information that the other woman was her mother (Austin 93), and opened the very first sentence with this narrative gambit: "What we did at Gettysburg, for the three weeks we were there, you will want to know" (3). Of course, the occurrences at Gettysburg were indeed of extreme interest to most Americans, but Woolsey bolstered intrigue all the more, creating a field of effective narrative magnetism between the anonymous, ambiguous speaker(s) and the audience whom she addressed directly.

The Sanitary Commission report gave a more or less populist justification for creating the commission: "The countless forms of popular sympathy growing more clamorous and persistent in their offers of relief as the war went on . . . bore unmistakable evidence of the determination of the American people to manifest in some way their direct personal interest in the soldier" (Stillé 82). Woolsey's narrative joined this popular clamor by situating a textual attraction in which the nurse narrator existed as a generative force fundamentally concerned with the relationship between the author and her audience. Garrett Stewart sees the literary moment of interaction between writer and reader as "*the* exemplary literary moment" (Stewart 12), and such an interaction made for successful political maneuvering for Woolsey, who used it to strengthen the cause and plump the commission's stores. She added lift to her address by delivering her message directly to the donor: "Some of you sent a stove (that is, the money to get it), some of you, the beef stock, some of you the milk and fresh bread; and all of you would have been thankful that you had done so, could you have seen the refreshment and comfort received through these things" (6). Reciting a list of supplies almost as emblems of writer-reader affinity, Woolsey allowed her audience to savor the knowledge that their contributions saw soldiers through illness and into recovery.

With such details she delineated the arc of connection with readers, and throughout the narrative represented many such connections between people black and white, and Northern and Southern—a tall order for such a short, almost brochure-length narrative. Woolsey ended *Three Weeks at Gettysburg* with an image embracing linkage, thanking her readership for saving soldiers' lives as the men waited for the "next train" (22). Recalling her opening description of the logistics of the hospital at one end, the railroad at the other, and the danger that the soldiers might fall through that gap between, she reiterated that the commission provided relief by closing the gap. She linked author and audience in a bridge of purpose so that comfort from home could be made available to the soldier in the field. Designing her narrative expressly for the purpose of reporting back to the community that the homefront and warfront remained connected and strong, she encouraged her readership to feel gratified that their donations had helped—and in doing this she spurred new donations.

Notwithstanding its many male leaders, the United States Sanitary Commission operated largely because of the exertions of women, and Woolsey took pride in the fact that she contributed to the good care received by soldiers. Women, the "small wheels," took pains to make all aspects of the operation run as smoothly as possible in the immediate aftermath of battle. Woolsey conveyed the impression that she and the other female relief workers at Gettysburg labored assiduously along with the women at home to attend to the needs and wants of their patients—or, as Woolsey wrote, "good hot soup was given all round" (6).

I think it would be more agreeable to you to come and see for yourself; one day is a pretty good specimen of every day, at least at present, so don your bonnet and jump into the cars with me. (23)

CHAPTER THREE

Julia Dunlap's *Notes of Hospital Life*

Women's Rights, Benevolence, and Class

Julia Dunlap's narrative, *Notes of Hospital Life*, occasionally mentioned in histories of Civil War nursing over the past decade or two, has been remarked on mostly because of its anonymity, the identity of the narrator remaining unknown until 2010. *Notes of Hospital Life* has received occasional comment also for the narrator's show of support for the working-class soldier; in the dedication, which began, "To the Privates of the Army of the United States," Dunlap gave a lengthy tribute to enlisted men for their daring, patience, self-sacrifice, loyalty, and noble example. Bypassing the work of officers to praise instead the work of military men of the lowest rank who often came from humble origins, Dunlap presented her work, from the dedication onward, as a narrative committed to class issues. The narrator's devotion to the working class and, even more so, her anonymity, have been the book's only claim to acknowledgment to this point.

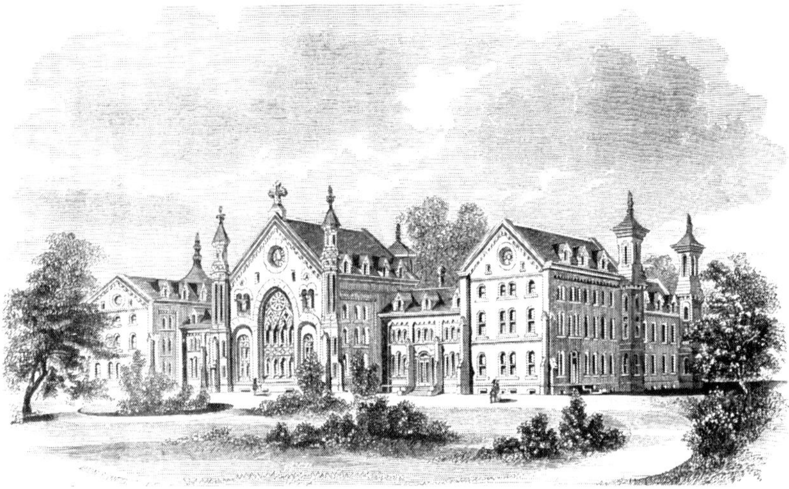

Sketch of the Hospital of the Protestant Episcopal Church, 1859

Courtesy of the Library of Congress

Dunlap's book can be read as a focused attempt to situate several substantial ideologies—those of women's rights, benevolence, and class issues—which affected Dunlap's practical decisions in her hospital work and structured the rhetoric of her narrative. Dunlap began *Notes of Hospital Life* with the "woman question," an issue of great importance to her, given the suspicion cast on women undertaking hospital jobs. Second, she embarked on the work of Christian benevolence or sympathy, which for her included nursing because the nursing program at her hospital was sanctioned by her church. Finally, Dunlap placed service to those of the working class as her first and foremost priority, a goal also in keeping with the mission of her church. Her personal interactions, however, did not always line up with her philosophical positions, and anonymity may have allowed her the leeway to explore such discrepancies.

SARAH JOSEPHA HALE defined "the woman question" in 1855 as follows: "the inherent right of the female to an equal participation with the male sex in all social, political, and religious offices" (753); Dunlap similarly voiced the right of women nurses to equal participation with male nurses in the field of Civil War relief work. Hale defined the entitlement of woman "to equal privileges with man, in the family, the church, and the state" (Hale xlii), and Dunlap adapted such ideas to apply to the right to equal privileges in her own circumstances. She attempted to counter the social disapprobation directed at female nurses when she presented, near the beginning of *Notes of Hospital Life*, a series of imagined voices, one after the other, as they criticized the nurse:

> "Women are not needed in these hospitals."
> "Depend upon it, ladies are a bore here."
> "The men are victimized." (18)

Aware of carping critics, Dunlap showcased the detractors' comments to accentuate the difficulties of working in an environment where female workers were disparaged. Characterizing the skeptics' voices as "bristling" and full of "indignant anger," she brushed off their animosity with tact and politesse to propose a refreshing idea: let the woman nurse leave the hospital if she is found to be other than helpful and other than able to supply a real need; however, if she is indeed useful to patients, "then let her go 'right onward,' unmindful of coldness, calumny, or comment from the world outside" (19).

Dunlap provided this solution of postponing for the moment the discussion of the ramifications of gender equality, asserting, "this is not the time or place to enter upon the great question of woman's mission" (20). In this she used the rhetorical tactics of deflection and indirection, as she seemed to suspend judgment even while arguing a point. In other words, by deflection she left the conclusion about women's rights to seem open-ended while by indirection she simultaneously finalized the parameters for acceptance of those, urging her readers to let the female nurse "go 'right onward'." Dunlap prioritized the war effort as the appropriate focus for the moment, but made it clear that she did not forget the "great question" of "woman's rights," tipping the reader off that the goal was still a noble purpose and that the purpose might be proved in nurse's labor itself.

In regards to the rhetoric of conversation, Dunlap took that tactic to the limit, assigning characters who aided Dunlap in allowing her readers to witness the female nurses' proficiency and to understand hospital life. First, Dunlap introduced her friend, M., so that she could craft a first-person plural "we," as Woolsey did, to share in the nursing experience. Arguing that the "we" was no "petty affectation of authorship" but the genuine situation, Dunlap insisted she and M. were actually friends and coworkers (38), but she made use of M. narratologically. Further, Dunlap assigned to the narrative another character, a listener, "C.," whom Dunlap knew well and to whom she intermittently addressed the tale of the memoir. C. was able to enter the hospital ward directly and experience the work of nursing, thus permitting the reader access by proxy. With the three women, M., C., and Dunlap herself, a triangle of identities was established to form a microcosm of community, anchored by church and hospital, that readers could visit.

Dunlap employed the rhetorical tactics of conversation and query in the brilliant first chapter, "Our Daily Work," which thematically recalled Alcott's chapter, "A Day." Here Dunlap structured her narrative with dialogue, and C. stood in for the reader: "You ask me, dear C., the usual question, when our work at the hospital is mentioned, 'What can the ladies find to do all day?'" (23). The question was "the usual" one asked by the curious and the critical, who apparently implied there was not much of import "the ladies" could have found "to do all day." Dunlap provided a quick response to C.: "I might give you the stereotyped answer, 'We receive and register the donations, give out and oversee the clothing, make either delicacies or drinks for the men who are ill, read to them, write for them, and try to make ourselves generally useful'" (23). Such an answer might be thought to close the case summarily in a positive compendium of the work conducted by women during the war.

Dunlap, however, added slyly: "This is the ordinary answer, but I think it would be more agreeable to you to come and see for yourself; one day is a pretty good specimen of every day . . . so don your bonnet and jump into the cars with me" (23). With this invitation she generated a narrative pull between writer and reader, urging, "What do you say?" (23). In an informal stroke Dunlap asked C., her reader's proxy, to accompany her into the ward, implying that she could fully validate the work of female nursing only if it was experienced firsthand. Her narrative solution was particularly apropos to the task, allowing her unobtrusively to address the material viability of women's work as she solicited readers to witness the various grueling and gratifying activities that comprised the nurse's daily schedule.

This approach gained its power from the immediate directive of the words, "jump into the cars with me," a phrase exhibiting an in-the-moment verve. She expressed such narrative energy at many cruxes, as in this: "Life in a hospital! When and where? Now and here" (17). Suggesting to C. that she would forget the little inconveniences of the trip—that the "sun is too scorching and the air too heavy"—and would soon lose herself "in more important affairs" (23), Dunlap proceeded in a step-by-step journey, instructing C. when they approached the hospital door to "acknowledge the guard's salute as we enter" (23). Dunlap took over once inside in the hospital as she instructed C. to observe this man here, that man there, "take a seat and look round you" (29), and "turn the key in that closet door" (30).

This stage-managing allowed Dunlap not only to argue the viability of women nurses, but to show them in action during difficult encounters. In the same chapter, Dunlap and C. stop to talk with one of the men, Jones, an "Irishman" with "a good deal of drollery about him" (24). Dunlap asked if he wanted anything, and Jones answered that what he wants she can't give, specifically: "it's some one to love that I'm wanting" (25). This was risky territory, as the interchange was exactly the kind of experience that critics of female nurses regarded as compromising to women's modesty and social standing. Dunlap, however, demonstrated her willingness to turn impropriety into humor with a ready response for the cheeky Jones: "you were right to say I couldn't help you, for unfortunately wives are not provided by Government" (25). With her resourceful answer Dunlap blocked potential disapproval and credited the ingenuity of women nurses, reassuring her audience that by dint of quickness and wit, women nurses were up to the task of protecting their reputations.[1] In this first chapter she provided a hands-on response to the question concerning what the ladies found to do in the hospital all day. To augment that point, Dunlap iterated at the end of the chapter that, "this day, just as you have seen it, is a counterpart of every day, not only of this week, but of the last three months" (37).

In answering C.'s question about what the ladies find to do, Dunlap subtly validated, with every subsequent mention of C. in the course of the narrative, the viability of female nurses.[2] She worked this option, indeed, to the point that eventually she could drop the apparatus of the character "C." altogether, and by prior narrative conditioning prompt the reader to insert herself into the text. For example, Dunlap spoke directly to the reader from the ward: "See how they are jammed together; on benches, on the dining-table itself, in the windows, and on every available spot, battered and bandaged, *wrappered* and wrinkled, suffering and smiling, in one promiscuous mass" (96). Dunlap found a way to continue without proxy of C. and use the second-person address directly to her audience with forthright, pressing, and inclusive diction.

DUNLAP VOICED HER worth as a nurse not only in a committed attitude toward women's rights, but in a committed discourse of Christian benevolence. Serving soldiers as she would have served members of her church or neighborhood, she attended to patients almost as she might have attended to a congregational community. She showed a personal interest in each patient, as is apparent in the chapter titles, often organized by the names of individuals: "Darlington," "Little Corning," "Gavin," "Poor José," "Robinson," and so on. Dunlap highlighted personal connections within the framework of the narrative, structuring one long chapter, "A Visit to the Wards," for instance, with explanations of particular patients' cases. By so arranging her narrative, she oriented herself as a social agent of fellowship and community-building in the hospital. That she could fortify the business of community-building in her workplace was unusual among the nurses studied in this project, in that Dunlap did not travel to a hospital site in a new city but instead worked at a hospital in the city of her residence. Probably writing initially for her church community, she exhibited a charitable outlook by which she bolstered her sense of neighborliness to extend the work of local church institutions into the wards.

As she did with women's rights, Julia Dunlap turned to the project of Christian benevolence with zest and ingenuity, attempting to allay the suffering of her patients at the same time that she sought to convert them to the Episcopal faith. She almost certainly would have been advised to follow this course by her church leader, Bishop Alonzo Potter, who in 1862 addressed the Diocesan Convention and spoke directly to the project of developing nurse charity: "Our camps and military hospitals are blessed schools for educating our benevolent affections and our capacities for charitable work" (Howe 58). Dunlap's willingness to convey the significance of that commitment to her readers was prodigious, albeit in the course of the memoir she became increasingly aware of the possibility that she could overreach with faith-based discourse. At one point, following her delivery of a sermonic Christmas lecture that occupied several pages, she confided to C. that she feared she had indulged in "tedious expression" (127).[3] Almost certainly, Dunlap would not have expressed such an awareness earlier in the narrative, because it was not yet necessary that she undergo alterations in perspectives; she spent the better part of the narrative defining such changes in outlook. The "tedious expression" comment clearly revealed Dunlap's continuing concern with articulating her message in a way that would be friendly to her listeners, comprising equally the soldiers listening to her Christmas sermon and the readers perusing her nurse narrative. Pursuing religious interpretations of the import of her labor, Dunlap at first privileged Christian dogma over informal talk in her interactions with soldiers, an approach that she came to see might not, at times, serve patients' best interests. A series of incidents caused her to reshape her method and modify a strictly Christian discourse potentially overwhelming to patients toward a more personally tailored manner that incorporated friendly, approachable talk.

For example, Dunlap adhered staunchly to a hierarchical view of Christianity when she conversed with a wounded soldier in the early chapter "The Two Armies." The patient asked her about an important visitor to the ward, whom he understood to be a military man. Dunlap knew the visitor was not a military man but the Bishop of Minnesota, but she declined to give that information to her patient, entering instead into a verbal riddle meant to instruct him. She implied the bishop was a military man, giving the details that he was a volunteer, had seen action, and had been wounded. The patient, intrigued, and not understanding that Dunlap was dealing in tropes apropos of the Christian ministry, asked her in which battles the man had fought; she surprised him when she replied that the man had never told a single person about any battles. Frustrated, the patient pointed out that if the man's service had been secret to everyone, no one could have known he was a soldier. Dunlap responded by claiming mysteriously that she knew the man's military service was a fact because she had also had the "privilege to be a Private in the same Army," though she was "not eligible for promotion" (45).

At this point the confounded patient interrupted her with the accusation that she was in effect toying with him, to which she responded by smiling and stating that she was simply trying to communicate with him in "a round-about way" (45). She alluded to a previous exchange between them in which he'd confessed he was trying to give up an unnamed behavior, most likely drinking.[4] Her comment made him feel exposed: his "color rose, but he said nothing" (46). Dunlap had attempted to give the patient a Christian lesson by drawing on a Christian trope, equating believers with soldiers, and thus demonstrating the military type of conviction it took to fight the dangers of unwanted behaviors or sin. The metaphor, however, fell flat, proving not a point of agreement between them, but a breaking point. Dunlap's attentions were off-putting to the soldier, who felt that her riddle made sport of him.

Though she thought she could reach him through the Christian soldier metaphor, she alienated him instead, possibly seeming to demean him for not giving up his vice. The soldier's reaction was marked; once he understood her point, he was embarrassed and angry, stating in no uncertain terms his aversion to mending his ways: "I'd liever go back to my regiment to-morrow, wounded as I am, than do what you want, though I know you're right, too" (46). He could hardly have given a more unambiguous message to Dunlap when he communicated that, far from being able to change his mind, she had changed only his willingness to engage with her. The upshot of her proselytizing was his total retreat from interaction: he pulled the covers over his head.

Dunlap had certainly been encouraged by the church to speak solicitously to patients about matters of faith, given that the Hospital of the Protestant Episcopal Church was her employment affiliation, and that the 1864 *Woman's Mission in the Christian Church*, an Episcopalian publication that promoted Bishop Potter's projects, predicated nurses' success in terms of their being able to bring soldiers in for confirmation: "The presence in another of the Government hospitals of the city, of refined and Christian ladies, co-operating with the chaplain, reveals the gratifying fact of forty soldiers and more brought in the course of the year to the solemn rite of Confirmation" (11). The church publication enumerated these soldiers won over to confirmation, reporting that there had been interest expressed also "in the elevation and improvement of those admitted to its walls" (11). Such a record of confirmation suggests that Julia Dunlap would have felt pressure to exert Christian as well as social ministrations in her hospital work.

At the outset of the narrative, Dunlap attempted to satisfy such expectations but ultimately moved from a tendentious approach to one more concerned with establishing fellowship through inclusive speech, from sermonizing to a more secular way of speaking. Mapping an unstated but profound transition in her approach to fellowship, Dunlap may have revised the notion of service by concentrating less on outcome and more on moments of interpersonal attention. In this way, the narrative proved to be as much about the success of changes in communication strategies as it was about the fact of conversion. Perhaps the most interesting facet of the above episode was the fact that Dunlap chose to tell the story about herself, electing to represent her actions in an unflattering way, including the fact that she had caused a patient to shut down to the point of pulling the covers over his head. She revealed her initial failure and also intimated that she might find later success if she changed her approach from church discourse to personal conversation.[5]

Dunlap wrestled with this difficulty throughout the narrative. In early meetings with soldiers she tended to frame a parallel between the conversion of the body to health and the conversion of the soul to faith. As a kind of template for her goals, she named an early chapter "The Contrast," so the parallel would not be lost. In "The Contrast," she distinguished Ennis, a soldier open to Christian teachings, from another, Jackson, a soldier altogether resistant. In the first case, the gentle, "childlike" Ennis began to improve from a severe illness, exhibiting an "eagerness to be taught—more especially upon religious subjects" (56), and in the second, the recalcitrant Jackson declined, brushing aside her ready help and steadfastly refusing to mend his ways, so that he remained a man "with unsteady step and bloodshot eye" (61). Ennis survived, turning into a "round, ruddy young soldier, looking particularly well in his uniform" (59), and Jackson never progressed.

Around mid-narrative, though, Dunlap underwent a sea change in her ministry, so to speak, as seen in her interactions with the patient Darlington and later with a crying patient in the corner of a ward, both of whom threatened to shut down on her as did the man who pulled the covers over his face. In the case of Darlington, others saw him as irritable and unapproachable, while Dunlap saw that he was suffering from a terrible wound and despondent over not being able to see his sister; he had only two modes of expression: either screaming in pain, or descending into severe depression. At this juncture Dunlap, beginning to amend her patient care to a more interpersonal dynamic, attempted to read the man's body language and tone of voice: "Anyone who had ever suffered realized that there was no crossness here; physical suffering, acute and intense, was written in every line of his face, sounded in every tone of his voice, and most earnestly did I long to soothe him" (83). In danger of dwindling health because of his self-imposed isolation, Darlington continued to fail, saying to Dunlap, "'Dear lady, please to go away, I am so very wretched'" (83). In response, she took action: "Without answering, I drew back, and laid my cold hands on his burning brow. His whole expression changed. 'You like it,' I said; 'I am so glad . . . '" (83–84). Dunlap tended to her patient in a gesture with the religious overtones of the laying on of hands but with the primary message of physical human contact. She chose to act with the certitude of spontaneous personal impulse and to heal by way of nurse–patient contact, and both were contented with the results.

In their next encounter, Darlington reinforced her approach, using signs to show that he wished her to repeat the treatment, and she responded that "'perhaps on this hot day, a little ice would be better; let me get you some'" (84). He exerted himself to speak, failed, and tried again: "'No! oh no! I said your hands were better than any ice'" (85). His response couldn't have been further removed from the response of the man who had pulled the covers over his head. Much of the impetus of the Darlington story derives from the fact that the two of them interacted primarily nonverbally, he gesturing and she responding with sensory comfort in a way that precluded Christian didacticism. At this point, Dunlap refused to fit the story of Darlington into a conventional redemption story.[6] The undoubted grist of the chapter was that she interacted with him in an individual, spontaneous, and authentic way, responding to genuine needs.[7] The scene of laying cold hands on Darlington formed the groundwork for Dunlap's ability to access moments of psychological and physical insight about patients. In subsequent episodes she resisted doctrinal explanations, at least at the core of her communications, despite sometimes tagging episodes at the end with scripture or Christian verse.

A final episode depicted this change in behavior in a surprising and charming interchange with a crying patient in the corner of a ward, in which Dunlap outstripped doctrinaire communication to favor the familiar, ordinary speech of spontaneous interaction.[8] Near the very end of the memoir, Dunlap told the story of a seriously ill soldier "crying like a child" (202), to whom she was alerted by the actions of a hospital dog named Dick. Dick pulled at her dress and gave her such "beseeching looks" that he seemed to be asking her to follow him. When she finally followed him, he led her to the upper corner of the ward that housed the most grievously wounded patients, where she saw the man who was crying. Dunlap may have exhibited, in responding to the dog, a willingness to step away from the top-down hierarchy of organizational dictates and act on her own recognizance, as she following the creature who seemed to have something to communicate to her.

The greater relevance of the tale, however, lay in Dunlap's interaction with the patient to whom the dog led her. When she saw the suffering patient she did not proceed immediately to his side but, surveying the situation first, gave herself time to evaluate it: "I stood a moment to take an observation — to make a sort of moral diagnosis before beginning my attack — to find out whether the man needed direct or indirect sympathy" (202). She comprehended that no two patients are alike, that different temperaments require different treatments, and accordingly observed her patient closely before acting.[9] Dunlap had developed detailed ideas for giving attention to specific personality types of patients:

> One [type] likes to suffer out all his suffering alone, to be as little looked after as possible. Another likes to be perpetually made much of and pitied, and to have some one always by him. Both these peculiarities might be observed and indulged much more than they are. For quite as often does it happen that a busy attendance is forced upon the first patient, who wishes for nothing but to be "let alone," as that the second is left to think himself neglected. (117–18)

After observing this patient, Dunlap decided that he was of the sort she termed nervous and therefore needed diversion. She walked up to him and related that her "assistant orderly" had informed her that she was wanted by him. He expressed surprise at her appearance, because he had not asked for help, and no person had been near him — only a dog, "'standing looking in my face, and wagging his tail, as if he were pitying me'" (206). At this point, Dunlap delivered her punch line, chiding the soldier for speaking "so slightingly of poor Dick," the very same creature that was the "assistant orderly" who informed her that the soldier wanted her.

In this encounter, the point was non-instructional and humorous, Dunlap valuing the moment with her patient for the sake of interaction and the betterment of his physical health. Her method of communication in the earlier chapter about the "Two Armies," in which the patient dismissed their conversation by pulling the covers over his head, had to do with her attempt to engage him in a kind of dialogic conversation that posed a riddle about Christianity. In the later case, Dunlap still used a dialogic model to question the soldier, and again pressed him to the point that he refuted her claim—that is, that "no person had been near him." The reader might fear that this interaction too will end in disconnection, but it did not, because Dunlap immediately changed to the interactive connection.

IN *NOTES OF HOSPITAL LIFE* Julia Dunlap also expressed support for the working-class soldier, as well as for the causes above. She took pride in aligning herself with the rank-and-file soldier and, as did other nurses, affirming the value of women nurses' service by reporting expressions of appreciation from the soldiers themselves. Dunlap watched the faces of patients as they noticed women nurses entering the wards, and stated, "I can truly say, that at all such times I have never, but once seen other than an expression of pleasure, and the warm greeting is apparently most sincere" (21).[10] One soldier, assuming that the soup served to him was scorched and tasted bad, refused it, until Dunlap explained that she had made it that morning with her own hands, with the flavoring he particularly liked. He responded, "'You made it, ma'am? The ladies? Then it's the kind I like'" (175–76).

Concerning working-class issues, Dunlap's bishop, Alonzo Potter, was from a Quaker background and staunchly supported programs to help working-class families. Dunlap began *Notes of Hospital Life* in accord with his principles, even extending her support of the rank-and-file to include a theory of art. She proposed that art and literature, in fact, relied on the contributions of the "everyman," repudiating the claim that only the privileged classes could conceive creative works. Basing her premise on an aesthetic that we would now call "cultural production," she declared in the first sentence of the Preface to *Notes of Hospital Life* that art did not rely on principles detached from society. The fact that the publishing industry had more or less collapsed during the war—with the important exception of literature written about the war—probably elicited a lamentation from one of her friends about such publications: "A literary friend said to me some time since, 'One of the greatest evils of this rebellion, is the manner in which it is tainting our literature, science, and arts'" (xi). Dunlap wanted to "break a lance" with this friend and defend literature published during the war as part and parcel of the work of the nation in totality. Evolving an aesthetic of artistic creativity that depended on the everyday life of the war, Dunlap wrote that hospital life had changed her:

> At the opening of the war I thought, with you, that the finer feelings of our nature were exclusively the property of the higher classes; but two years' experience in a military hospital, where men appear mentally as well as physically in "undress uniform," has shown me the utter fallacy of such a theory; and now I do not hesitate to affirm that I have seen there as much unwritten poetry, tender feeling, aye, and love for the beautiful, as I have ever witnessed . . . (xii)

She used the phrase "undress uniform" to designate the physical state of patients but also the condition of being able to appreciate unadorned art, heralding an aesthetic that resulted from lived experience. Dunlap endorsed art that refused to put on airs, commended the beauty of unself-conscious expression, and venerated the army private as a person of good taste in his own right. Fahs notes that "two years as a nurse in a military hospital" had shown the narrator the fallacy of thinking that only the upper classes have access to finer perceptions (116). Dunlap's lengthy dedication to her book, "To the Privates of the Army of the United States," praised a democratic literature that included "daring in danger; patience in privation; self-sacrifice in suffering." She crafted the preface to mitigate any hubris in her own text, a choice made for similar reasons when she opted for authorial anonymity. In the most succinct formulation given by any nurse narrator about the job of writing, Dunlap affirmed the simplicity and unassuming quality of her composition: "These notes were jotted down as the incidents occurred; they are a simple statement of facts simply stated" (xiii). Committing to the text written and read by the every-person of military service, she extolled the working-class soldier as the major cause of *Notes of Hospital Life*.

Dunlap's views didn't always come easily, though. Rhapsodic about men of the common ranks in her introduction and preface, she did not carry through consistently with that tone when it came to certain challenges in interpersonal exchanges. Her positions on class, like those on Christian sympathy, were works in progress, and as she changed she came to confess her own shortcomings, showing herself, again, remarkably willing to "tell" on herself. For instance, early in the narrative she encountered a man she perceived as being "of very low origin, bad habits," and about whom she confessed with shame, she felt an "unconquerable disgust" (69). Later, though, despite her "disgust," she gave him an opportunity to undertake an action of generosity toward another soldier by going to fetch some desired food; the man with bad habits validated her trust by carrying out the task. Though the defense and commendation of the working class was her theme, including her insight that "the human heart is the same all the world over" (173), she at times had to grow into that theme.

Especially in the chapter "Poor José," Dunlap assured the reader that she championed the working-class man and immigrant by detailing a scene of complex social interactions whereby she became involved in helping the title character. She urged the reader to challenge the intentionally ironic epigraph, "'But these men have no feeling'" (128), demonstrating unequivocally that working-class men absolutely have feeling. Dunlap enjoyed talking with the enlisted man José, a "self-made" Spanish immigrant, whose family had fallen on hard times. José had endured destitution, his family's eviction from their house, and his wife's mental illness, and was becoming distraught about his children's foster care. Boarding his three children with a neighbor who had stopped sending him news of them, he missed his sons Juan and Henriquez, but most particularly his favorite, the four-year-old daughter, "little Rosita." Dunlap offered to seek information about the children for him, though her readiness was quickly checked when she learned that the children were lodged in a Philadelphia neighborhood of disrepute. Dunlap's reaction to this news was emphatic: "I started, and shook my head. 'That is impossible; I could not go there . . . it would not be right'" (131).

At this juncture her eagerness to do good met her class bias and sense of propriety, resulting in a tangle of motivations. Dissonance underlay many philanthropic motivations, as many nineteenth-century proponents of charity owned unacknowledged reasons for undertaking philanthropy, including the desire to vaunt their character in lofty contrast to the outcast character of the persons they aided. An additional complication, as Susan Ryan points out, was that "a too-thorough identification between helper and helped risked a degree of social leveling that most donors would have resisted, as well as the loss of the destitute other against whom the benevolent defined themselves" (19). Dunlap realized she risked social leveling in visiting the neighborhood, but the redoubtable José continued to urge her, saying, "'God will protect you'" (131), a Christian argument she surely would have had trouble dismissing. Perhaps most of all, the leader of her church, Bishop Potter, favored hands-on aid for those in need, given that he had "supported a parish . . . visitation of unchurched working-class families" (Pritchard 152).

Dunlap had only indirect knowledge of the neighborhood in question, though she knew of such a neighborhood by way of an author's account. She equated the poverty-stricken Philadelphia neighborhood with a neighborhood described by Elizabeth Barrett Browning: "Suffice it to say, a certain account of 'St. Margaret's court,' in the matchless poem of Aurora Leigh, was before me, stereoscoped into life, never again to be mere word-painting" (132). An educated woman, Dunlap had to perceive the real-life setting before her by projecting Elizabeth Barrett Browning's epic poem, *Aurora Leigh*, onto it. The task of trying to find José's children was so entirely outside her experience that she needed the literary corollary, which included a rouged woman, a woman with a lascivious mouth, the presence of cholera, cramps, spasms, oaths, a mildewed wall, dropping plaster, and more:

> Within St. Margaret's Court I stood alone,
> Close-veiled. A sick child from an ague-fit
> Whose wasted right hand gambled 'gainst his left
> With an old brass button; in a blot of sun
> Jeered weakly at me as I passed across
> The uneven pavement . . .
> —(*Aurora Leigh* 89)

Scenes of extreme indigence were common in nineteenth-century novels and popular magazines such as *Godey's Lady's Book* and *Harper's*, in works by Rebecca Harding Davis, Harriet Martineau, Charles Dickens, and Harriet Beecher Stowe, among others. Dunlap had undoubtedly read some of these, which were sure to cause discomfort to middle- or leisured-class readers, but had no doubt responded with benevolent sentiment, never imagining she would confront people living in such conditions, even in her own Philadelphia, the second-largest city in the country at the time.

Dunlap entered the neighborhood and found a combination grocery/apartment where the children lived, the surroundings including "suggestive-looking sausages" hanging from ropes, "gnarly green apples," and other unappetizing foods, all serving to "crowd the little, low, dirty counter, behind which stands the live stock of this interesting apartment" (132). A particularly indelicate pun, Dunlap used "live stock" to designate the inhabitant who oversaw the children: "something between a crone and a hag, with coarse Irish features, loose dress, hair hanging down, and apparently guiltless of any tending of either comb or brush since she had attained maturity" (133). Dunlap further denigrated the woman for mispronouncing the name of José's son, Juan, calling him "*Jewann*" (133). Betraying her bias against Irish immigrants, an intolerance rampant in nineteenth-century America, Dunlap most likely drew from countless harsh anti-immigrant texts and cartoons to create the above description, showing her difficulty, again, in registering the inhabitants as anything but literary; that is to say, she had a hard time seeing them as real people.

As soon as she laid eyes on Rosita she knew her at once as José's daughter, a perfect little girl who embraced Dunlap and curled up in her lap at the mention of her father. Dunlap recognized the "stain" of poverty on Rosita but made clear that it could be seen optimistically: "A large stain of the dirt in which she was living, rested on one cheek; but it seemed merely a shadow bringing out the bright tints beneath" (134). Nonetheless, Dunlap also seemed to script Rosita as culturally "other," given her "large, liquid, Spanish eyes," "tangled black curls" (134), and wearing feathers in her cap like a Native American. When Dunlap asked Rosita what she would like to say to her father, the girl gave her one of the feathers, which Dunlap asked for as a material sign to show to José that the family bond held.

When she returned to the hospital to visit José later, Dunlap witnessed an overjoyed father joined by his three children. Such a familial image allowed her to end the chapter with a reminder of the ironic epigraph that had launched it: "'But these men have no feeling.'" As Dunlap walked past the happy family group, José held up a feather for her to witness in passing, the token signaling reunification. While it referenced what Dunlap would have seen as the boon of charity work, in that she had been able to restore three children to their father, at the same time it preserved the hint of ethnic difference that some benevolence workers needed to ameliorate the threat of social leveling.

A problematic element of the sequence remained the suggestion that the Irish-American woman caring for the children did not have the faculties of "finer feeling."[11] To point out this problem is not to say that Dunlap's dawning open-mindedness concerning class was altogether vitiated because of her bias in other areas; very little of a person's experience can happen in only one ethical register at a time. All of the nurse narratives were written during a time of tumultuous social change, and *Notes of Hospital Life* focused, in turn, on each way station in social understanding along the road for a relatively privileged white woman attempting to make sense of ethnic and class changes. Dunlap turned the rhetoric of Christian theology to the work of helpful interactions and, though flawed, she tried to improve herself, experience by experience, and to talk to her reader about it in a surprisingly honest and increasingly familiar way.[12]

As regards class open-mindedness, near the end of the narrative Dunlap recorded a remarkable exchange with a working-class soldier. She at first felt uncomfortable with the soldier's outspokenness but stayed to hear him, and by staying may have prompted his further candidness, for he then spoke in extraordinarily unambiguous words about the savage politics of military conflict, about officials and working-class soldiers in the Civil War:

> I'll just tell you how it is, in this war. We're all a set of ten-pins, stood up to have balls sent at us; along they come, and down we go. No matter, get another set; but still, it may save Uncle Sam to mend the

> broken ones, and use them again; so the menders come along, pick you up, feel you all over, and see if you're worth mending; if so, you're patched up, and stood in your place again. (186)

That Dunlap chose to record this scathing speech at all is remarkable. She probably permitted herself the liberty because the soldier spoke the words as prelude to a further point in which he commented respectfully on the power of compassion exhibited by a particular doctor. The soldier commended the doctor as a man remarkable for his sympathetic powers, and who was as a result,

> different from the other menders: but it's all in his eye— . . . it says, "You're flesh and blood, you are, poor fellow? and I'm sorry to see you twisting about with pain like that, and it's all a bad business, this same, so it is." (186)

The soldier lauded the doctor who tended not only to the body but the heart, affording relief to the whole person. Dunlap marveled at the man's wisdom when he said he "feels better for a whole day" after seeing that doctor, feeling better not even for the kind act or kind word: "For none of these; but merely for a look—a glance of sympathy!" (187) She proved brave in recording this soldier's trenchant assessment of the business of war and insightful in conveying the power of the doctor's personal concern for his patient. Because she was willing to stay in that interpersonal encounter that was at first uncomfortable, she proved honest with her readers and willing to accept unusual perceptions.

THERE ARE SEVERAL historical documents that lead us to verify Julia Dunlap's identity and substantiate her community alliances. The biographical trail leads from the narrative's place of publication, Philadelphia, to Bishop Alonzo of Philadelphia, who vouched for Dunlap in the narrative's introduction, to the Episcopal Church of Philadelphia, to the bishop's pet project, the Episcopal Hospital, on Front and York Streets, in which Dunlap worked. Julia Dunlap chose to omit her authorial identity, as did Georgeanna Woolsey, and while the identity of the latter surfaced relatively quickly, Dunlap's was obscured until 2010. Most likely, Dunlap chose to remain unknown as a marker of feminine modesty. She probably wasn't concerned that her ideologies would offend the smaller circle of her church members, given that Bishop Potter supported all three of the ideologies examined above, especially that of helping the working class. She may have been concerned, however, if she imagined that her narrative might reach a larger circle of readers outside the congregation, where she might have been seen as prideful in claiming individual agency in relation to the community causes of the church. In his introduction to her work, Bishop Potter saw the anonymous Dunlap as a modest woman author who spoke only as a service and at the insistence of friends.[13]

Because Dunlap's identity has been so recently revealed, we will trace the provenance that led to verification of her name, finding authentication in the materials that associated her nursing work with the hospital in Philadelphia. The starting point is Bishop Potter, who initiated Dunlap's book with an introduction lauding her discernment of the working-class soldier's character, "the delicate tastes and noble sentiments that often possess those whose hands have been hardened by toil" (ix). As Bishop of Pennsylvania from 1845–1865, Potter was a proponent of temperance, abolition, and "'hospitality to the poor,'" which he thought "should be the motto" of every church (Howe 212). He founded the Episcopal hospital at Philadelphia . . . as well as, "if not the first, certainly among the first, of those experiments out of which has grown the establishment of Apprentices' and Young Men's Lyceums" (Howe 63). As mentioned above, his projects no doubt influenced Dunlap in her concerns for the common soldier.

The Episcopal hospital was linked with the Episcopal church, both under Potter's leadership, and given their circle of associations in both institutions as well as his contribution to Dunlap's book, it is likely that they knew each other. Potter's introduction covered either directly or obliquely all the major concerns addressed in her narrative: the "woman question," acknowledging the public need for women nurses; the ideology of Christian sympathy, accessing Harriet Beecher Stowe and her famous phrase "right feeling" (vii); and class equality, about which he stated that the narrator's heart is one "which can feel that which makes all the world akin—which can see that labor does not degrade, but rather elevates those who pursue it in the true spirit" (ix).

Dunlap would have been conscious of performing what the 1864 publication of the Episcopal Church of Pennsylvania, *Woman's Mission in the Christian Church*, referred to specifically as "missionary work." These notes corroborated the success of women's work: "Owing to the presence of ministering women the comfort of the patients has been increased, their recovery promoted, better order maintained, and a general air of cheerfulness and brotherly kindness has prevailed" (*Woman's Mission* 14). The notes authenticated too, the basic democracy of decency inherent in the working class: "Under woman's influence thus exerted, rude, rough men, who at first rejected proffered kindness, were soon softened and completely changed; manifesting deep gratitude to their sympathizing friends" (15). As we have seen, she was expected to perform the work of religious instruction so as to bring patients into the church for the purpose of conversion.[14] Dunlap operated, at least in the early parts of her narrative, according to the expectations of those who made her service possible, catering to church members who were likely the first readers of her book.

Immediately after the release of *Notes of Hospital Life* this same Episcopal Church of Pennsylvania reviewed it:

> That graceful and captivating little book, "Notes of Hospital Life," which has just issued from the press, and whose scenes are laid in one of the Philadelphia asylums for the soldier, illustrates the spirit of many scores of workers in this department of charity, while it shows the delicacy and tact of womanly ministration and its marvellous [*sic*] power for good over the suffering. (*Woman's Mission* 11)

The reviewer commended the book for showing the benevolent spirit "in this department of charity" within the church. Albeit anonymous to the world at large, Dunlap was likely known to some church members, and it is reasonable to infer that she envisioned, at least at the start of the project, that she would write about her nursing experiences almost exclusively to this target audience of congregation friends and acquaintances.

The book was published by J. B. Lippincott, also in Philadelphia, who "capitalized on the hunger for war stories by publishing *Notes of Hospital Life*," which sold moderately well (Schultz 228). Given this larger audience, Dunlap may have decided on anonymity, a choice her culture upheld as her prerogative, because she was concerned about seeming too outspoken. Grappling with issues of the woman question, sympathy, and social class, all of which reflected high-profile American cultural issues of the time, Dunlap took complex, changing positions, which may have "played" better within the context of the church audience than outside it. Quite possibly because of the sensitive nature of her personal challenges in experimenting with doctrinal discourse, which she would not have wanted the outside world to interpret as being critical of the church, she elected namelessness.[15] Easley sees a paradox in gender politics when considering female anonymity: "Ironically, it was the suppression of individual identity through anonymous publication that enabled the development of new definitions of women's political subjectivity and liberal individuality" (*First-Person Anonymous* 3). With the option to manipulate authorial identity in nineteenth-century culture, women could articulate views that might otherwise have been difficult to claim. Dunlap made herself potentially vulnerable by engaging in the mission of caring for many different types of soldiers, pondering the nature of the type of care she gave, and demonstrating that preconceived ideas were not always useful in some of the individual encounters she had.

The respect accorded the choice of anonymity can be seen by the fact that in late 1893, almost thirty years after the publication of Dunlap's narrative, a writer for a volume of *Book News: A Monthly Survey of General Literature* spotlighted *Notes of Hospital Life* but remained firm in protecting the author's identity, despite the fact that the writer possessed the information, stating, "We do not feel at liberty to give the author's name" (21). Not everyone, though, had been so scrupulous. Two years after the narrative was published, Linus Brockett included an excerpt in his popular 1866 volume, *The Camp, the Battlefield, and the Hospital; Or, Lights and Shadows of the Great Rebellion*. The story, "Robinson, the Wounded Soldier," a chapter from *Notes of Hospital Life*, told of a soldier who whistled to keep his mind off the severe pain caused by war wounds. Brockett's press, the National Publishing Company, based in Philadelphia (as well as Chicago and St. Louis), took the liberty of naming the author of the story as "Miss Dunlap," introducing the piece as follows: "Miss DUNLAP, a Philadelphia lady, who devoted herself with great assiduity to the care of the wounded soldiers in the hospitals, which were so numerous around that city, has related some incidents of her experience in the hospitals in a most charming volume, entitled 'Notes of Hospital Life,' a work deserving of much wider circulation than it received" (316). Dunlap also received recognition in an 1864 *Boston Recorder* reprint of a segment of her work with the story of Dick, the hospital dog, under the title, "The Four-Footed Orderly"; the *Stroughton Sentinel* reprinted the same under almost the same title.

One last publisher proved even more forthcoming than Brockett. Sarah Josepha Hale, editor of *Godey's Lady's Book*, included Dunlap's first and last name in Hale's ambitious 1874 compendium of the distinguished women of all time, grandly entitled *Woman's Record; Or, Sketches of All Distinguished Women, from the Creation to A.D. 1868*. Hale designated Dunlap as one of these women:

> Among the enduring works we name also "Notes on Hospital Life," by *Miss Julia Dunlap*, of Philadelphia. It shows that refinement of feeling and culture can light up even repulsive scenes with the delicate beauty of Christian sympathy. All who read the book will understand better how love of country and faith in God can sustain American women in their duties. Its pages are "full of spirit, of wisdom, and of right feeling"—so says the late Right Reverend Bishop Potter. (Hale 900)

In fact, Hale wrote the same commendation earlier in 1868, in *Godey's*, prefacing it by stating, "The war literature was mostly ephemeral," and presenting Dunlap's narrative as a remedy to that (*Godey's*, October 1868, 358). As Hale asserted, Dunlap wrote an enduring narrative of Christian sympathy and most likely undertook exactly that goal of working in the service of Christianity. While Hale thought Dunlap wrote a narrative of Christian sympathy, she failed, however, to see that Dunlap set that goal at the beginning but proceeded to write a book that along the way found a less dogmatic framing of that Christian sympathy. Perhaps because of her anonymity, Dunlap managed to create a narrative of candid account and acute reflection as she contended with her own nineteenth-century cultural biases. As she would say, she wrote along with those working-class men who expressed themselves informally in "undress uniform," telling her story by way of jotted-down notes in "a simple statement of facts simply stated."

. . . the 'word' which 'makes men free' . . . (67)

CHAPTER FOUR

Elvira J. Powers's *Hospital Pencillings*

Travel, Dissent, and Cultural Ties

Of the nurses studied here, Elvira Powers traveled farthest from home and served in some of the most varied and demanding jobs, journeying south to Nashville, where she worked in a hospital, a smallpox ward, a school for freed children, and a Southern refugee institution for the homeless. Her stay in Nashville occurred during the time that General William Tecumseh Sherman captured Atlanta in September 2, 1864, his maneuvers at points circumscribing her excursions. On April 28, 1864, Powers canceled plans for a trip from Nashville to Huntsville, Alabama, because "Sherman closed the way" (*Hospital Pencillings* 61), and several months later, on September 22, she again scuttled plans, this time from Chicago to Rome, Georgia, because "Sherman had issued an order forbidding any except soldiers going beyond Chattanooga" (89). She left Nashville to save the life of a nurse friend whom she accompanied back to her home in the west (now the Midwest) to recuperate, and thereafter transferred to one of the largest hospitals during the war, Jefferson Hospital in Jeffersonville, Indiana, a hub because of its access to the Ohio River. There she became the matron of a ward at which, among many duties, she worked briefly in the gangrene tents. Along the byways of her journeys, Powers sometimes spoke her mind frankly about the operations of hospital affairs.

From the very beginning of *Hospital Pencillings*, Powers borrowed from women's rights rhetoric, dedicating her work not to the privates, as Dunlap did, but to the female workers who served privates and other soldiers. The lengthy dedication showed an unapologetically gendered approach: "To our loyal countrywomen, who, at home, in camp, field, or city hospital, by purity, true womanliness, and that labor which is worship . . . have contributed to the aid, comfort and consolation of our sick, wounded, and dying 'braves in blue.'" She valorized the troops, of course, but foregrounded their female caretakers, to include women working in the home as well as in the field and hospital. Powers continued to underscore gender in the preface, asserting that "the inducement which the author had for offering this little volume to the public was the fact that at the commencement of this four years' war, it was next to impossible to obtain any information upon the subject of the duties and trials of women nurses in military hospitals," and that "the little which appeared was read with exceeding avidity" (Powers v). Initially there had been a lack of reportage, though many accounts of female nursing had set a corrective to that by the middle and end of the war, and by the time *Hospital Pencillings* appeared in 1866.

Little is known about Elvira Powers, except that she wrote *Hospital Pencillings* and was a member of the Universalist Church. Assertive about fair treatment, Powers may have derived some of her tenacity and fortitude from her association with the politically liberal church, in which she was trained in theology. A Universalist retrospective, *Fifty Notable Years*, reported that she went to Canton Theological School as part of the New York Convention, but had to leave the school a half-year later because of "ill health" (Adams 255). Her Universalist association probably influenced her choice to submit a segment of her narrative for publication in the *New Covenant*, a Universalist newspaper based in Chicago. Powers suggested that because part of the narrative in the *New Covenant* had "'attracted much attention'" (vi), the book based on those contributions would garner yet more attention for women's labor. Initially recording events in her diary, Powers doubtless arranged and revised diary notes for the newspaper segment, then afterwards compiled material for a book. The *New Covenant* boasted as its assistant editor the noted nurse Mary Livermore, and as editor her husband, Daniel Livermore. To publish in the *New Covenant*, Powers may have pressed her connection with Mary Livermore, given that both had served as nurses and that both were members of the Universalist church.

Powers also attempted publication in another venue, contributing a sketch from her narrative in Frank Moore's *Women of the War*, which appeared anonymously; finally, she "persuaded Edward L. Mitchell of Boston to publish the whole" narrative (Schultz 230), *Hospital Pencillings*. Powers's correspondence with Frank Moore shows that she also wrote to him about the poor quality of reportage about women nurses at the war's onset. Offering for his consideration a very brief, admiring sketch of Annie Bell, matron at "Hospital No. 8, of Nashville, Tenn.," where they met, Powers suggested that there had been not only a scarcity of news, but an appreciable amount of misinformation about women's service:

> [Annie Bell] was at first opposed by her friends in her desire to enter a hospital, they probably entertaining an idea quite prevalent in those days & shared by myself & which kept me from going for two long, regretted years. This mistaken idea was relative to the nature of the duties required & the supposed character of those who discharged them. But like another she was so pressed with a sense of the duty required of her that she could scarcely eat or sleep until she obeyed the call. (Moore papers 5–6)

Powers emphasized Bell's conflict in wanting to serve at the same time she feared that female nursing was disreputable; interestingly, Powers noted that she herself shared this uncertainly and as a result missed out on the chance to serve during the first two years of the war, a source of disappointment to her. She referred to Annie Bell, but also obliquely referred to herself in the phrase "like another"; retaining modesty by not naming herself directly, she proclaimed her patriotic fervor and readiness to serve.[1]

This readiness derived precisely from fervent commitments to women's rights and abolition, which attendance at theological school and association with her progressive church fostered. These causes employed emblematic and transformative discourses to change consciousness and sometimes politics, and given that she lived in this time of swiftly changing social issues, Powers often looked to rhetoric to leverage meaning. She constructed narrative scenes in the belief that the precisely chosen word could clarify a complex cultural situation and generate and justify political action. For instance, Powers used the word "Emancipation" as a benchmark term. In response to acquaintances who had told her that on arriving in the South she would become pro-slavery, she reported having just the opposite experience, especially when she witnessed racial tension caused by a white man in a black church, which caused her to redouble her belief in Emancipation. She described "Emancipation" as a kind of gospel, claiming that it "is the 'word' which 'makes men free'" (67). To contextualize the power of this word, she further invoked a stanza from Julia Ward Howe's "The Battle Hymn of the Republic": the gospel "read by the 'watch-fires of an hundred circling camps'" (67). The word "Emancipation," as valued in the combined rhetorics of abolitionism, Christianity, and American liberty, formed the gospel for this nurse's mission, the linguistic site at which the war's "circling camps" found their purpose. To examine the ways in which such powerful terms shaped Powers's narrative, we will examine travel, dissent, and the cultural linkages she developed in *Hospital Pencillings*.

POWERS MADE AMPLE USE of the nurse narrative strategy of travel in concentrated anecdotes in the beginning of her memoir, describing her movement to the south as a means to show the difficulties women nurses faced and so create a sympathetic sisterhood between writer and audience. In Powers's memoir, travel was also a kind of touchstone for guiding readers to cultural openness, as she met people of diverse races and regions. Quick-witted and broad-minded, she described journeys in the Southern and Western theatres of conflict by depicting other travelers, expressing the difficulties of transit during wartime, and detailing local color and items of regional interest. Not surprisingly for a word lover, she recorded the names of new flowers and fauna on the train ride south, at many turns asserting that she was after all, a "Yankee schoolma'am," (140)[2] and evincing a dogged desire to educate herself: "Here was a chance to add to my rather meager stock of knowledge in natural history" (4). For example, when she and her companions passed near Mammoth Cave, she mused about the cave's blind fish and commented on redbud and mistletoe, from which she "secured specimens" (60). In detail worthy of Henry David Thoreau, Powers described a magnolia blossom: "It is in shape and size something like the African lily, and grew upon a tree the size of the common apple. It is of a peach-blow hue upon the outside and white within, and with the mingled fragrance of the roses and lemon" (70). Among the multitude of flora, she did not omit the cotton blossom,[3] but only in that instance did her botanist's interest turn political: "King Cotton rather disappointed me in his personal appearance, presenting rather a sickly and woe-begone look," as compared with Yankee wool, the appearance of which was more "imposing" (100).

Powers's observations typified the purpose of proving the nurse's mettle through the hardships of travel. Like Alcott, Powers offered tales both anxious and humorous as she communicated the difficulties of approaching a new place of employment. Journeying by boat, hack, and train, Powers left Cincinnati on April 1, 1864, with her friend, Miss O——, another woman nurse, and met up with an escort, Mr. R. from Louisville. Miss O—— and Mr. R. proved game travel companions, as for instance when Mr. R. teased the two women by asking them if, when they nursed soldiers, they would attend only to "the good-looking ones" (2), to which the women rejoined that they would attend only to the "ministers, doctors, lawyers, or editors" (3). Continuing such banter, Mr. R. attempted to ready the women for medical service by telling them a story about a woman nurse who, upon asking a patient if she might comb his hair, received this reply: "Yes—you—*may* . . . but it will be the thirteenth time today'" (3).[4]

Powers interspersed travel anecdotes with issues of women's rights in a lively way, as for instance, when her party transferred to the train at a chaotic depot. At this depot they entered a kind of reverse-gendered world in which females held power because they received preference in seating; in response, men hustled to curry favor so they could pose as escorts and thereby gain a seat. Noting that each man scurried to find a lady to "take him under her care" (7), Powers commented that the women were "in too great demand altogether" (6). In one particularly comical instance, a man helped a woman carry her box onto the train in hopes of being able to stay aboard, and when he succeeded, handed the woman's box out the train window to a waiting friend, who in turn used it to secure his passage onboard, likewise handing the box out the window to yet another man. Such a travel scene accomplished the dual purpose of drawing the reader in with humor and showing the dedication of the nurse as she moved so far from her familiar home.

As they traveled farther south toward Nashville, the train passed a military encampment, which Powers noted had been set up on an inferior site instead of being set up on a fine green sward only a few rods away. She remonstrated that "any officer who would compel his men to pitch tents where those were ought to be levelled to the ranks" (8). Delivering her pronouncement decisively, she included the consequence she saw as fit punishment for the officer's folly: demotion. This vignette proved the mettle of Powers's character as it anticipated the determination with which she would approach the need to make judgments as a nurse, to include some judgments that included dissent.

She started to see a change in the landscape when she surveyed "fortifications, stockades, rifle-pits, and mounted cannon at the bridges" (8), until there was no doubt they were traveling through occupied territory, as evidenced further by the "burnt fences and the levelled trees" (8). At this point Powers saw a black man who was not a refugee but a soldier:

> In the deep cut passes one sees suddenly the picturesque figure of a negro soldier, far above upon the heights, who with shining uniform and glittering bayonet stands like a statue, guarding the portals of liberty (8).

To cue the import of the sentence, Powers switched the first-person subject of the sentence from the personal "I" to the more formal "one." She viewed the soldier in "the deep cut passes," emblematic of the cultural recesses to which the enslaved person had been consigned by force, now with the promise of arising and standing "far above upon the heights." The soldier wielded a "glittering" weapon, wore a "shining" uniform, and guarded "the portals of liberty," a phrase that refocused the meaning of the war from preserving the Union to freeing enslaved people as the best means to protect American freedom. Despite using the sentimental and unfortunate word "picturesque," Powers portrayed a man who owned the power, agency, and honor due his position.[5] The figure of the black soldier guarding American liberty, in the early pages of the memoir, provided an imagistic authority that depended upon a mixture of the discourses of abolitionism and patriotism.

AFTER SHE ARRIVED AT THE Nashville hospital, Powers uncovered neglect and misuse of power in the actions of some hospital officials. When it came to dissent, Powers leaned very heavily on the rhetoric of abolitionism as the underpinning for her actions. Once on a course of dissenting action, she was not easily deterred: "Being by nature and birth an outspoken New Englander, and having inhaled freedom of speech from the breezes which blow from the hills of the 'Old Bay State,' I fancy it will not be very easy becoming initiated into this phase of military service" (20). Gathering discursive power from the illustrious history of the Massachusetts Bay colony, she upheld her right to take action, associating the Bay State with its rich heritage of civil disobedience and antislavery protest.[6,7] Powers tended and revised a cultural narrative of free speech inherent to American liberty, invoking the Bay State to rely on its history of dissent, which allowed her early in the narrative to oppose a corrupt chaplain.

It is important to clarify that the word "dissent" is used here in its broadest sense, to include the disagreements with regulations and behavior in the hospital and the strategies undertaken to address any given disagreement. Incidents of dissent configured significant portions of Powers's memoir as she found herself in conflict with powerful figures, including a chaplain and a physician. Both the chaplain and physician cases appeared to be interlocked, escalating to a crisis that probably contributed to her dismissal. Later in the narrative, Powers would come to buttress the recounting of conflicts with a newfound confidence that may have helped her regain footing when she transferred to Jefferson General Hospital in Jeffersonville, Indiana; she arrived in Indiana ready to read the dynamics of interaction in her new hospital and prepared to develop a fresh and penetrating model whereby she could comprehend workplace politics and communications.

In Nashville, though, Powers first dissented against a Nashville chaplain who showed gross negligence in his failure to visit the sick and dying patients under his aegis. While she declined to divulge the chaplain's identity, she did name one of the patients who died on his watch.[8] Chaplain S. shirked his duties regarding the patients in his wards, specifically Ward 1, where "two to four boys are dying daily, while the Chaplain has not been in to speak to a single sick or dying boy for two weeks" (19). Moreover, Chaplain S. disregarded his obligation to write condolence letters to the families of the deceased, which was a serious breach. As Powers earnestly asserted, "it was his duty," and also "common humanity would dictate that it be done" (19), and on these points her audience would have fully agreed. Faust points out that such condolence letters were of paramount importance, in that they "may have served in part as . . . a way of moving symbolically out of the meaningless slaughter back into the reassuring mid-nineteenth-century assumptions about life's meaning and purpose" (31). Perhaps the fact that Powers had trained for the ministry added to her righteous anger in censuring his neglect. She decided to write condolence letters in the chaplain's stead, a task nurses frequently undertook when no chaplain was available. In this case, the job was his, and he disregarded it.

But Powers went further, lodging a complaint about the chaplain's behavior and submitting a grievance to more than one authority. She was surprised to find herself repulsed by the system, "given to understand by more than one Christian minister, that the expression of indignation was considered a bad omen for my future success in hospitals" (19). Not only did the authorities ignore her protest, they thought it indicated that her behavior needed correction and they advised her to pretend that she did not witness misbehaviors: "'people here . . . must learn to see and hear all manner of evil and wickedness going on around them, and be as though they saw and heard not'" (19). She found that "more than one Christian minister" passively condoned the shiftless chaplain's behavior, but even worse, she began to suspect that the attitude might be systemic.

The situation escalated when, in a second incident, Powers seemed to enter an even larger network of officials who apparently upheld the status quo to protect their own. She found herself summarily threatened with dismissal without explanation, a situation that caused her to offer a caustic aside to her readers that she liked this "military style" of justice because it saved one "the trouble and worry of defending one's self" (63). Suspended in uncertainty concerning both the nature of her infraction and identity of her accuser, she later discovered the specifics through the grapevine: "the terrible crime for which I was tried, convicted, sentenced and banished" (63) was that of having used infelicitous language in advocating for a patient because a surgeon found it undermining to his authority. In other words, her "crime" was her choice of language. Powers had tended a patient who begged for a mustard poultice, a request she couldn't honor without permission, given that men nurses were assigned that particular duty. She found the surgeon and asked him, "'Doctor there is a patient in the third tent below, on bed No. 9, who is in great pain and wants a mustard poultice. Will you see if he needs it? If so, I can make it'" (64). The doctor responded by giving the patient something for pain, but not a poultice.

Powers' analysis of what she called, ironically, the "grave charge" (62) leveled against her stemmed from a linguistic scruple inherent in the different meanings of the word "want." The doctor "used the word *want* for *need*, so that when I said the man "wanted" it [the poultice]—meaning he had *asked* for it, he interpreted it so as to convey the idea of my assuming the responsibility of saying 'he needed it'" (65). Even though Powers and the doctor both had the patient's well-being at heart, each possessed a different lexical understanding that impeded their ability to work together toward a shared goal. Further, Powers intended the use of the word "see" when she said, "see if he needs it," as a request that the doctor check the patient's condition, while the doctor apparently construed the word to mean the imperative, as in "see to it." Admitting she might have acted with "unusual brusqueness" (64), she added that her approach arose from an uneasy mix of feelings, including trepidation—she had heard that "some physicians were offended even by a request" (64). As Sizer comments about the same episode: "The degree of conflict that could emerge over both word choice ('want' and 'need') and inflection (her 'brusqueness') suggests the tension simmering between surgeons and nurses" (207).

Powers came to suspect that her termination was caused by tension with both the physician and the chaplain, which she believed "it would scarcely be policy for them to mention" (65). The final step in sealing her dismissal was probably her act of committing her disagreement to writing, as she sent Chaplain S. a note of reminder that the men would like him to visit them in the ward, but did not receive a reply or see him in the ward. On the same day, though, she noticed him "engaged in pitching quoits" for a leisurely half-hour: "I knew he had not been in to see a single sick or dying soldier in my division since my stay, nor preached a funeral sermon for the many who had died in my division alone" (65). She added that he was well-paid for these services he did not perform. Powers's reminder to the chaplain constituted an action she was "certain had something to do with my departure" (65). When she expressed her disagreement in writing, Powers engaged in her most audacious tactic of dissent—a high-risk maneuver of outright confrontation in a penned communication directly advising an authority to do his job.[9] Both gestures—informing the doctor about the mustard poultice and writing the chaplain a reminder about his duties—involved her use of words as the act of transgression.

Elvira Powers moved on to another assignment at a smallpox ward in which she again discovered grievous ineptitude in a medical establishment and felt strongly that suffering could be prevented.[10] The smallpox ward, located outside Nashville, was notable not only for its size but its diversity: "In these tents are about 800 patients—including convalescents, contrabands, soldiers, and citizens" (42). The large facility was also notable because, with the exception of physicians' wives, only one other woman beside herself worked there. Powers reported smallpox episodes with a frank realism and lack of squeamishness, taking note of the "unsightly, swollen faces, blotched with eruption, or presenting an entire scab, and the offensive odor" (42).

In the smallpox ward she discovered that many of the patients assigned to the facility had measles instead of the more deadly disease: "*Sixty cases of measles* were sent to this [smallpox] hospital in *one month*," she related, adding drily that such a fact can "impress one with a sense of the importance by the medical faculty of distinguishing between the two diseases" (43). Much later in the narrative she reported the same gross misdiagnosis and mis-assignment of a man deemed to have smallpox, who was carried twelve miles on a bitterly cold day, without being dressed, to a smallpox hospital. Powers had suspected that he had measles, and later found that she was right, but by the time the patient was correctly sent to the measles hospital, he had taken cold, lost consciousness, and died. In a noteworthy moment of decrying institutional inefficiency to her readers, she asked poignantly: "He has fallen a victim to what?" (171).

Though Powers never voiced her outrage about the smallpox misdiagnoses to authorities, she grew more confident in her instincts as a medical worker who could direct her rhetoric to the audience who would hear her—her readers—and she used the discourse of patriotism to advocate for patients. With the pleading interrogative, "He has fallen a victim to what?" she implied that a man's suffering and death could have been prevented by an alternate course of rooting out neglect and bolstering workplace efficiency. In the case of the smallpox ward, she did not act but wrote instead, resisting injustice by informing others through her narrative. This method of social dissent through writing had been especially popular for several decades in prevalent American newspapers and magazines, which featured such authors as Harriet Martineau, Charles Dickens, Herman Melville, and Rebecca Harding Davis, who decried unfair industrial labor conditions and other social problems. Many women learned to speak out through protest and, as Jacqueline Bacon points out (specifically about abolitionism), many white women "often negotiated these seemingly contradictory requirements" of being "feminine" and "rhetorically authoritative" by strategically combining the two to "challenge and expand traditional assumptions of their society about gender" (112). Some nurses did this for the rights of patients; from Alcott to Wheelock, the woman nurse engaged in written speech as a potent means of voicing demurral and potentially effecting change. Alcott, for instance, after witnessing how roughly a surgeon treated soldiers, felt a powerful urge to give an otherwise respected surgeon some of his own medicine, and even while she was carrying out his orders she was "cherishing the while a strong desire to insinuate a few of his own disagreeable knives and scissors into him, and see how he liked it" (71). She didn't intervene but she did involve her readers, and *Hospital Sketches* succeeded in reaching sectors of her audience in time to prompt "a public outcry about conditions for soldiers" (Eiselein, Philips 140). Powers, working and writing at the end of the war, did not have the latitude to change Civil War medical practices, but could inform readers about medical and institutional injustices. Railing against the hospital's incursions into the nurse's right to register opinions on patients' health, she pitted her fervid Massachusetts civil disobedience against the instances in which the hospital allowed negligence.

While Powers began her service by taking the risk of penning disagreement directly to the chaplain, she seemed, after being compelled to change jobs, to refine her tactics, and to report infractions to her audience instead. In her later service in Indiana, she may, paradoxically, have actually increased the effectiveness of her workplace interactions by altering the mode of her dissent. Ultimately, Powers's dismissal in Nashville became a mere pause between jobs that permitted her a kind of sabbatical to spend modifying her approach to institutional conflict. As an aside, during Powers's transition between Tennessee and Indiana she met Mrs. Mary Ann "Mother" Bickerdyke, a famous nurse and large personality, probably the most storied of assertive women during the Civil War. Having been relieved of her post, Powers sat down to write Bickerdyke a request for another hospital position, to be surprised when the woman herself showed up in Nashville, en route to the front to ac-

company Sherman's army.[11] Bickerdyke was celebrated for her audacious ability to procure goods and services for soldiers, despite the obstruction of bureaucracies.[12] While Powers saw Bickerdyke's personal style as overly blunt and confrontational, she also undoubtedly learned from her strong example, recognizing her as "a perfect hero in the army, among sick soldiers" (75), where their gratitude proved the highest ethical standard for justifying an action. She also benefitted from the Bickerdyke model when she moved to her next post.

Powers next found employment at a large institution, Jefferson General Hospital, in Jeffersonville, Indiana, where she utilized a slightly new form of address to facilitate workplace interactions, all the while retaining her self-proclaimed "Yankee schoolma'am" temperament and progressive New England outlook. This new address fit the more comfortable labor conditions at Jefferson Hospital, where Powers enjoyed the position of nurse matron, which allowed, at least in her ward, an increase of mutual respect between physician and nurse: "How kind they all are. I receive nothing in my ward from the surgeon down, but the greatest respect and consideration. Some of the ladies can get no assistance, but those in our ward are ready at all times to help" (138). Here she tailored a different course of action when she felt the need to disagree, using communication tactics more intricate than those in her Nashville encounters.

The course Powers took still depended on a shrewd understanding of language, as she had demonstrated before in analyzing the words, "want" and "see"; now she honed that understanding to interpret the way signals function within a workplace system. Regarding communication in an organization, Michael Huspek observes that a member of an organization "must be expected to bow to the rule-dictates of specific institutionalized discourses as a requisite for being understood" (12). Powers employed her verbal finesse to "read" the rule-dictates of her workplace, just as she would "read" any other communication. For her to be able to speak truth to power, she would have to be cognizant of these dictates and thus engage in a work discourse that allowed her to be heard, "as a condition for speaking 'the true'" (Huspek 12). Specifically, Powers deciphered the rule-dictates among military officials in her ward at Jefferson

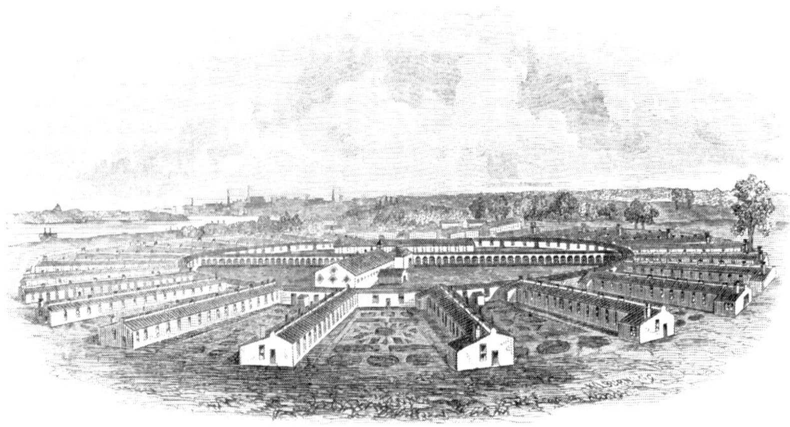

Jefferson General Hospital, Jeffersonville, Indiana
Elvira Powers, *Hospital Pencillings*

Hospital during a ward inspection which revealed to her the workings of a military hospital in which the female civilian nurse served.

The ward inspection that helped her to understand her position in the workplace happened, by accident, to include her. This event, occurring about a month after she was assigned to the new post, centered around the word, "Attention," at which she was alerted to a sudden military ritual: a bugle sounded, attendants arranged themselves on either side of the doors, and a group of officials entered, including the surgeon-in-charge, "the executive officer, the officer of the day and our own ward surgeon" (131). Powers noted the array of command trappings in the officers' bearing of gold leaf, green sash, gilt stripe, buttons, and epaulets: "When the surgeons appeared, at the word of 'Attention!' from the ward-master, each man rose to his feet . . . and the Inspectors marched swiftly through the ward" (131–132).

Unable to discern the proper protocol required of her during this inspection, she felt confused as to whether or not she should rise from her seat to acknowledge the presence of the top-ranking officials: "I was uncertain about what should be my own position, having thought nothing about it" (132). In terms of organizational discourse, the word

"Attention!" signaled a coding of rule-dictates Powers was not yet able to "read." Her solution was to take two opposite actions, in a kind of half-and-half approach; she rose from her seat, but after the inspectors went the length of the ward to the bathroom and turned around, she sat back down. Comically, the fact of her sitting down then elicited signs of homage from the inspection group, as she "was honored by a lofty bow from two or three of the dignitaries" (132). The loftiness of the bow, and the fact that only some but not all of the officials executed the bow indicated they, too, were slightly flummoxed about proper protocol concerning female nurses.

After this incident Powers didn't wait to sort out confusion as she had in the Nashville hospital, but went directly to a ranking official. Comprehending that the hospital system "expressed" its speakers, so to speak, she wanted transparency as to how the system's gestures (bugling, appearing, marching, ranging at doors, rising, sitting) indicated rule-dictates. Powers approached the surgeon because she was "determined to know whether I ought to rise or not before next inspection day" (132). He responded that only soldiers need rise—"and you are not a soldier, are you?" (132). Her position was a double-bind in that she had the duty to abide by military standards of job performance, even though she was outside the chain of command; by way of response to that quandary, the surgeon accentuated that she was defined by a negative—that is, she was "not a soldier." The inspection, initialized by the word "Attention!" and coded by the structure of operations, revealed the organizational contradiction, which made it absurdly possible for Powers to choose to stand for half the ritual then sit for the other, possible to locate herself as an agent both inside and outside the system. Powers situated and secured her institutional position when she inquired about this contradiction, directly alerting her superior to the workings of the organization and prompting him to articulate the nurse's role, thereby clearing new aisles in the corridors of power for the female nurse. Powers illuminated a kind of rhetoric of actions in the telling of her tale about upholding women's rights within an organization. Her actions allowed her to prepare herself to gain the leverage to speak "the true."

Powers's act of defining the rule-dictates helped her to accrue a modicum of power in confronting incompetence and wrongdoing in the hospital, especially as concerned bureaucratic red tape. Powers inveighed against red tape and was able to fight against it in part because she understood workplace systems, and so perceived red tape as something that clogged the "body" of the institution. Unsurprisingly for a healthcare worker, she used an anatomical analogy, suggesting that red tape, "in its rightful province forms the firm ligatures which keep in their proper places the different portions of the social and military systems" (78), but in its wrongful place does damage, as when the military body was "sometimes distorted from its original use, and made to subserve the interest of petty underlings and unprincipled officials" (78). If the connections were abused, they caused systemic sickness in the body of the institution itself, which caused devastating results for patients. The unscrupulous "underlings and unprincipled officials" of many institutions, as she pointed out, saw it as their prerogative to tell other workers "that all sin and high-handed wickedness which is wrought in high places, must be 'winked at'" (78). At Jefferson Hospital, she was able successfully to expose bureaucratic negligence and the collusion of officials in misdeeds, whether the obstructionist actions of an angry clerk, an unrealistic rule regarding the diet list, or a regulation targeting unmarried women.

Powers used women's rights rhetoric and interpreted most cases as instances whereby the system unfairly "expressed" and supplanted the position of women, as for instance when she exposed the ludicrous operations of a clerk in the course of Powers's attempt to procure a mattress for one of her patients who suffered for lack of it. Foiled by regulatory snags, Powers attempted to donate her own mattress to the patient, only to provoke the angry clerk to respond that he wanted to "give the wardmaster a piece of his mind for letting a *woman* interfere in the matter" (127).[13] In another example, a new regulation was instituted to systematize the removal of women's involvement in the preparation of the diet lists. An order was sent to all the wards, declaring that only surgeons could make out the diet lists, "as it was feared in some instances the lady nurses were allowed to make them out" (127). This order resulted in doctors and nurses collaborating to sidestep the order so they could continue in the same practice they always had, except for now they needed to put in the extra work to cover up the fact. In effect, they dissented by using the tactic of interpretation of a rule, which allowed them to follow the specifications if not the intent of the rule. One doctor, for instance, coped with the new regulation by copying over Powers's list in his own handwriting, another by asking her to copy and add his signature to her list, and yet another by requesting that she dictate the diet to him while he wrote, so the order would be in his script, "thus complying with the letter of the order" (127).

Yet another example recounts the surgeon general ordering that no lady nurses should be allowed in the hospital except those who were the wives of soldiers. This preposterous order was met with humor, Doctor C. and Mr. Bayne joking with Powers that they would have to hunt her up a husband so she could stay. Apparently having a particular candidate in mind, they asked her if "'red whiskers will be a serious objection'" (173). By reporting this humorous interchange Powers revealed the ludicrous quality of the attempt to discredit women by defining them only as they existed in relation to men, as wives. The regulation showed another version of the complex position the woman nurse occupied, which was, again defined by a negative: Powers was not a soldier, and in this case, not a wife. With this order, however, events intervened to have the last word: Powers reported the regulation on February 11, 1865, and by May 9, 1865, the war was over, and at the end of the final six months of her postwar stay at Jefferson Hospital, not a single doctor or nurse remained except for Elvira Powers.[14]

BECAUSE NURSES serving during the Civil War were institutional workers with no well-defined role, hospital assignments were sometimes halting and lapses common, and as a result women nurses at times took on obligations in addition to those at the hospital. Assigned to the Tennessee hospital facility and then summarily dismissed because of her dissent, Powers continued to live in Nashville before she found the position in Indiana, and during this interim briefly formed acquaintanceships within the diverse community in the area. During this time she communicated and forged ties with people of different demographics of the American population, showing local cultures underrepresented in Union narratives, such as urban Nashville freedpeople and southern Tennessee refugees.

In representing Nashville freedpeople living in territory occupied by the Union, Powers spoke as an abolitionist whose rhetoric had crossed the 1863 divide delineated by the Emancipation Proclamation, from the fight for antislavery to the fight for social equality, a discursive crossing that by 1866 she had made somewhat more successfully than Alcott and Woolsey. The Nashville freedpeople population led lives that differed greatly in degree from the lives of refugees displaced to the North, who were often homeless and at the mercy of unfamiliar circumstances. By contrast, the Nashville urban population lived in more or less longstanding, intact black communities. Powers taught at a "colored school" of 400 students, including some "really astonishing" students, like a seven-year-old girl who could "read fluently in the Fourth Reader," and a twelve-year-old boy who had been to school only nine months but could "read in the Third Reader" (62). Powers's admiration for her pupils inspired her to comment that "one might now not only exclaim with Gallileo [*sic*], 'the world *does* move,' but add and we *move with it*" (63). As a teacher she perceived that the world was changing not only in the minds of her students but in her own as well, and as an abolitionist who had reoriented herself to a new cultural understanding prompted by the Proclamation, she perceived the vitality of a diverse American citizenry in the making. Powers also held private classes for two black children, a job that included teaching a young boy, Peter, to spell the word "occupy" (115–16), a resonant word given their position in Tennessee as individuals protected by the presence of the occupying Union army.

Powers's connections in the black community opened up opportunities for other associations, such as her attendance at the "colored preaching," held in the same building as the school. After reporting on the stylish clothing and fine appearance of the congregation, she emphasized the adept use of discourse during the sermon. This was the meeting, by the way, that inspired her to speak of the eminence of the word "Emancipation," as the word redoubled her sense of mission, and which she passed on to her readers so they could likewise be roused to a renewal of the sense of cause. She wrote, "I'm getting to believe that the day when the Emancipation Document was set forth, was that of which it is said 'a nation shall be born in a day'" (66). She additionally wrote, concerning "the 'word' which 'makes men free,' that it would forever strike the manacles from the oppressed bondsman" (66–67). When she spoke of this "word," she hinted at the Christian scripture in which God can "make men free from danger" (Daniel 6:27).

Most importantly, in this church scene Powers identified a potent rhetoric initiated not by herself, the white narrator, but by the black preacher. In the metaphorically rich sermon, the black preacher concentrated on the biblical story of Peter taken away by the angel "as easily as though 'his chains were made of wax and a lighted candle was held beneath them'" (67), so that the melting of Peter's chains left the soldiers powerless to recapture him. Upon hearing this story of escape and liberation "one old man laughed outright, a joyous, grateful laugh" (67). The justice and joy of the gospel was intrinsic to the congregation's sense of liberty and their belief in the efficacy of abolition.[15] Powers's role in conveying this discourse was that of being aware of a freedperson's Signifying use of language as a rightful representation of black emancipation.

Powers was proud of the black community in Nashville,[16] but had few corresponding feelings for the white Southern refugees, whom she perceived to be shiftless—at least partly because she saw them, given her regional background, as being raised to believe "labor a disgrace" (36). These homeless Southerners were extremely unfortunate: "the filth, destitution, misery, and ignorance which exist among that class of poor whites who have fled from starvation . . . must be witnessed to be realized" (36). Powers's depiction of the refugee home was not for the faint of heart, for she included grisly details, particularly concerning the suffering of women and children. By contrast to much Northern war literature that concentrated on the physical suffering of soldiers, Powers highlighted in this section the suffering of the Southern civilian population, reporting on children in rags, an abandoned woman with consumption, a woman addicted to opium, a young woman with a disease that was probably syphilis, orphans without even a distant family member to be contacted, and a particular fourteen-year-old boy with measles who was illiterate and thus unable to locate surviving relatives. She seemed to cast aspersions on the morality of the white refugees whom she reported as sufferers of addiction, sexual disease, and family dissipation. In another case, she told the story of three young girls who lived through the devastation caused by armies from either side crossing their property. First the Union troops looted and destroyed their home, after which the Confederate troops advanced and looted their home, until once again the Union troops marched through, at which point the girls were finally removed to the refugee home.

On a very different note, when Powers left the South and returned to hospital work in Indiana, she attended another demographic, the Native American, even less mentioned in narratives. She briefly encountered two men from Michigan, possibly from the Ojibwa or Pottawatomie tribes, both of whom had recovered their health enough to be granted furloughs, but were stranded because the army had left them unprepared for January travel from Indiana to Michigan. One of the men had no coat and no money because he hadn't remained at the facility long enough to receive his two months's pay, and also no descriptive roll was available to requisition clothing for the journey. Powers found one flannel shirt left from the January stock and asked for socks and flannel drawers from the Sanitary Agent who stipulated that they could be had only in extreme cases. Powers pleaded the urgency of the case and received the articles for the soldier, commenting to the reader that he was "not of the copper-headed but of the copper-colored race" (156). The pun, perhaps overwrought by our standards, would have been liberal in Powers's time, marking her disgust for the "copperhead" or Northerner who pitted himself against the Union cause, and proving her contrasting esteem for the superior Native American patriot. The other Native American man spoke only a couple of English words and held in his possession a letter written to whomever he might encounter along the journey home, explaining his situation and asking that he be helped. Powers and the soldier spoke by signs so that she could convey to him the importance of retaining the letter for the voyage. She called an ambulance to take both men to the depot, only later to learn that the vehicle never arrived and the men had to walk a mile in muddy conditions to get to the train. Though she was unable to help as much as she wanted, she fought red tape—the institutional rule-dictates that she had learned to finesse so that at times she got results. She procured the supplies and assistance in some cases, as she worked for various demographics.

Elvira Powers, a staunch supporter of women's rights, abolition, civil disobedience, and progressive Christianity, brought her Massachusetts heritage to various locales in Tennessee and Indiana, experiencing remarkable interchanges with disparate populations. She spoke her mind in the attempt to bring justice to neglected soldiers and to foster their morale. Officials' reactions toward nurses improved to some extent during the course of the war, as can be seen in a final 1866 report for the Indiana Sanitary Commission. Dr. William Hannaman, who probably did not know Powers, asserted a dramatic change in physicians's attitudes, as Peggy Seigel reports: "Praising the service of Indiana's Civil War nurses as he had done for the past three years, he [Hannaman] wrote, 'No soldier upon the battlefield deserves more credit for bravery [than nurses]; none proved themselves truer patriots,'" (24). Powers encountered that attitude in her service across the country, as well as its opposite, and little by little found more efficacious ways to maneuver around and against obstructive protocols as she confronted the obloquy aimed at the competence and viability of the female nurse. She constructed an identity for herself within the discourse of the hospital workplace so that she could perform most effectively the job of augmenting her patients's well-being and her own.

Nothing before us all the day but wounded men; men at every step you take. (76)

CHAPTER FIVE

Anna Morris Holstein's *Three Years in Field Hospitals of the Army of the Potomac*

The Dead Line

Anna Morris Holstein worked most often in extreme situations. Her service encompassed four major locales or campaigns: the Battle of Antietam in 1862, Gettysburg in 1863, the campaign of the Army of the Potomac in 1864, and Annapolis Barracks, where she nursed returned prisoners of war in 1865. Holstein organized these locales in her narrative's four chapters, to create *Three Years in Field Hospitals of the Army of the Potomac*, a forthright chronicle of some of the Civil War's most gruesome fields of suffering. Very likely, Holstein saw as many sick, wounded, and starving soldiers as any nurse who left a record of service. Not usually confined to a hospital building, she worked with her husband, camping near the front "within sound of musketry and cannon" (30), where she could sometimes "plainly" see enemy soldiers (31), ate bread four- or five-weeks old, and slept in a tent with pine needles for a floor (27). At one point she carried a concealed sword: "I wore under my coat a belt, and carried the costly sword belonging to it under my dress. A civilian, as my husband was, could not do so without danger of arrest, while I would pass unnoticed" (36). Holstein could conceal the sword because her position as a female nurse remained undefined, rendering her outside the realm of expectations.

Before the war, Holstein and her husband, William H. Holstein, lived a comfortable life as a "wealthy and prominent couple living in upper Merion, Montgomery County, Pennsylvania" (Hall 45), until 1862, when William went to work for the Sanitary Commission.[1] Like Dunlap, Holstein hailed from Pennsylvania, was published by J. B. Lippincott in Philadelphia, and mentioned a "beloved" Bishop Potter; given the mutual connections, the two women may have known of one another. Both Dunlap and Holstein chose anonymity, or in the case of Holstein, near anonymity, with only the name "Mrs. H." on the title page of *Three Years*. Claiming modesty, Holstein asserted that she wrote primarily for friends: "To preserve some slight memento of them [war events] for friends at home, was the primary object of these notes: to gratify the same persons are they now grouped together" (v). She published, however, in a major press, Lippincott, which advertised the book at least twice in *The Round Table*, a New York weekly. The memoir received reviews, too, all of which indicated an audience wider than simply that of "friends at home." Schultz points out that because Dunlap's narrative "sold well enough," Lippincott subsequently published Holstein's *Three Years* (228). Other than these similarities, Holstein's outlook held little in common with Dunlap's, for the two Pennsylvania women worked in extremely different venues, Dunlap remaining in her home city of Philadelphia, and Holstein frequently on the move in dangerous locations.

Holstein provided an unflinching report of the horror and enormity of battle, such raw, extenuating circumstances probably contributing to the creation of a narrative more fragmented than most.[2] The fragmentation mirrored the transitory nature of her experience and the devastation caused by the number of suffering patients she witnessed. Using strategies common to the nurse narrative, Holstein first expressed her

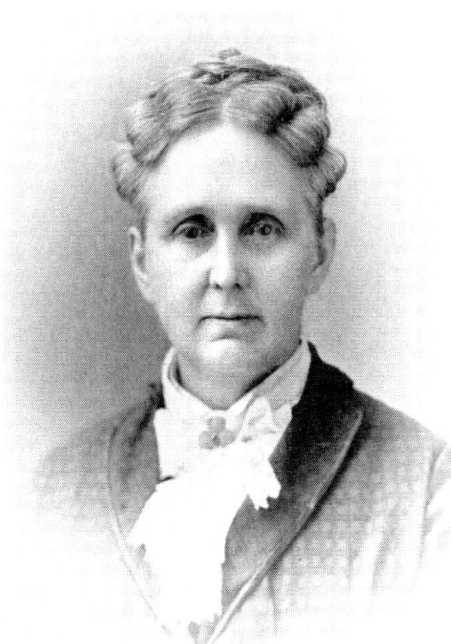

Anna Morris Holstein

MOLLUS Massachusetts Civil War Photographs, United States Army Heritage and Education Center, Carlisle, PA

motivation for volunteering and the difficulties of travel, and continued to use travel throughout as a way to fortify a conversational link with her audience; she depended more than any of the other narrators studied here on the rhetoric of indirection and deflection. In *Three Years*, Holstein created a writer–reader bond when she addressed these nurse narrative features: nurse travel and motivation, nurse dissent, linkages (between races and between the homefront and warfront), and finally, more controversially, the interrogation of war suffering.

HOLSTEIN BROACHED THE FIRST of these narrative strategies, nurse travel and motivation, by attesting in an initially surprising scenario that she was less than eager to join the war effort. In fact, she "declined" to join six other women who had decided to serve, admitting that "the idea of seeing and waiting upon wounded men, was one from which I shrank instinctively" (10). Instead of exhibiting Alcott-like panache about the prospect of traveling far from home, she confessed fear, though she still accomplished the purpose of the narrative strategy of travel in that she prepared readers to feel sororal compassion for the nurse, to empathize with her discomfort and natural aversion to taking a job initially seen as inappropriate for women. Holstein chose at first to stay home, with "all loyal women of the land" (10), and contribute to the war effort from within the community. She made clear her motivation, which was simply the need to satisfy the "irresistible impulse *to do, to act.* Anything but idleness, when our armies were preparing for the combat" (10). Though at first she contributed to the war effort domestically as her husband left to help at the front, when he returned soon afterwards "with the sad story that men were actually dying for food, home comforts and home care . . . I hesitated no longer, but with him went earnestly to work in procuring supplies of food, medicine, and clothing" (11). The soldiers' need for provisions spurred Holstein to become directly involved, and once at work she realized, on first seeing wounded men in the hospitals, that nursing was a calling, stating that "*this* is the work God has given *me* to do in this war" (11). Speaking at first with a culturally sanctioned femininity, Anna Morris Holstein resisted the nontraditional job, but later recouped her energies to justify the purpose of female nursing, able to claim that the impetus arose from "the purest motives of patriotism and benevolence" (11). She took a stance both modest and exultant to testify to her solid character, skillfully framing of the complications of women's roles to set up a bond of understanding with her readers.

Holstein's initial reluctance to attend to wounded men was a complicated response, which she used to convey a kind of modesty that she might share with her female readers and thereby galvanize the audience bond, as for example in this passage:

> It was *impossible* to be an idler while this gigantic struggle was in progress. The current of swiftly passing events had, all unconsciously, drifted me to this point; I yielded to its force, and commenced this additional labor as part of the work which came unsought. There was not the least recognition of *self* in any part of it; had there been, it would have been impossible to have gone on with it." (54–55)

She loaded these sentences heavily with words that avoided personal agency and posited fate as the prime mover—words such as *impossible, current, swiftly, events, unconsciously, drifted, force, unsought*—attempting to exhibit her deflection of individual needs and her acceptance of the huge forces of conflagration. Suggesting that service was not to be construed as self-serving or self-aggrandizing, she employed the rhetoric of indirection to the utmost, eliding almost completely the relevance of personal identity and decision-making to emphasize the sweep of action in which one woman played a miniscule part. Through this rhetoric she prompted the reader to decide for herself the respectability of female nurses.

Yet another feature of nurse narratives included the adoption of a rhetoric from a contemporaneous social movement to justify gestures of dissent. Though the narratives of Powers, Bucklin, and Wheelock presented numerous occurrences of dissent, Holstein's narrative recorded only one, and that one brief. Perhaps she found fewer causes for dissent because she, unlike the other women nurses studied here, was accompanied by her husband, a circumstance that doubtless shielded her from some of the difficulties of being a woman working among military men. Her situation may have mitigated possible derision from officials who instead deferred to Holstein out of respect to her husband; indeed, she portrayed her experience of being the sole woman in camp in extremely positive terms: "I have been for weeks the only lady in a camp of seven hundred men, and have never been treated with more deference, respect, and kindness than when thus situated" (55).

Holstein's one example of dissent revealed the rhetoric of indirection and deflection, shown also by her temporizing of the event afterwards. Her dissent, though short-lived, carried an intrinsic drama that announced the scene's centrality and importance, given that her antagonist was "one of our best and most experienced surgeons" (67), and given that she depicted his using a method of wound dressing inferior to hers. At White House on the Pamunkey River in Virginia, Holstein and other relief workers became almost overwhelmed by the thousands of General Benjamin Butler's wounded, many of whom needed immediate attention. One soldier in particular, so feeble that he leaned on another's

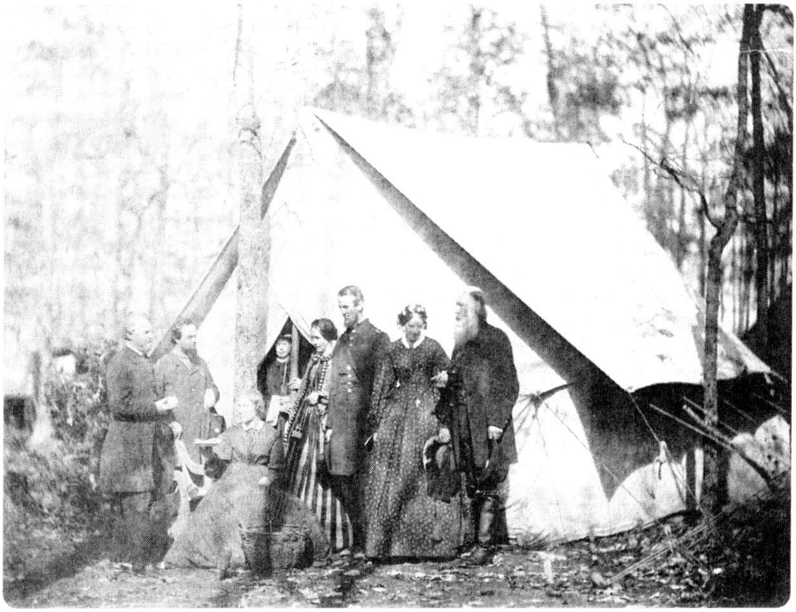

Anna Morris Holstein (fourth from right) and husband, William H. Holstein (far left), Gettysburg, United States Sanitary Commission, 1863

MOLLUS Massachusetts Civil War Photographs, United States Army Heritage and Education Center, Carlisle, PA

shoulder, braved his way forward to ask if she would dress his wound, which he described as "'in offensive, bad condition, filled with creeping life!'" (66). The particular task he requested was generally reserved for male wound dressers, and Holstein admitted, characteristically, it made her feel uneasy as she "shrank from the task, but persevered until it was nicely cleansed and dressed" (66–7).

The story turned suspenseful at this point because, on finishing the job, she realized that "hundreds of others, reclining upon the ground, were intently watching the process" and that, "eager for their turn, one after another came slowly up, with the same query from all: 'Would the lady dress their wound?'" (67). Holstein, the lone woman, surrounded by hundreds of men with more medical needs than she could possibly fulfill, was approached by one "rough-looking Irishman," with a "fearful-looking" head wound. Holstein chose to report that the patient expressed disgruntlement with the doctors' treatment and asserted that he preferred her treatment to the theirs's, saying "'he could bear any pain I gave him, if the doctors did not dress it'" (67). Yet a further point of intrigue arose when the doctor himself, who happened to have been watching the scene develop, intervened:

> . . . observing what was going on, [the surgeon] came to my relief, and, to the utter dismay of the poor fellow [with the head wound], took the sponge out of my hand to show me how much too tenderly and carefully the work was done; at every movement of the sponge in his hand, the soldier's head bent and shrank beneath the touch, but not one word of complaint escaped him; as the doctor moved away, his [the patient's] thanks were *not* for the kindness shown him, but that he [the surgeon] was *gone*, and that my unskillful hands would now finish. (67)

Needless to say, a trenchant irony resided in the deflective phrase "my unskillful hands," in which Holstein stated with seeming modesty the superior method of feminine attention, in a rhetoric of disclaiming judgment while actually arguing a point, as Bacon earlier identified (159–62). Relying on the stereotype of the rough Irishman, Holstein impressed upon her reader the point that even the most stout and uncomplaining of soldiers preferred compassionate and even tender medical attention, which might offer a kind of healing in itself. Holstein underscored the fact that the surgeon behaved with an overly blunt manner, edging into abuse, because in that case he used his position not primarily to heal the patient but to punish Holstein. He signaled his resentment of her action by discharging his anger against the body of the hapless soldier.

Holstein engaged in an act of dissent when she chose to dress a wound she knew was not technically part of her job description; afterward, however, she seemed to offer a retraction, retreating before the "regular dressers" as they came to start their work. She described herself as "the one who had usurped their office [who] gladly disappeared among the heaps of edibles which filled the shelter nearest us" (67–8). Characterizing herself as a usurper, she withdrew to the field kitchen or storehouse to deflate her presumption of power but, still, she chose to show the thanks of the soldiers, an act which superseded all else: "the sincere, heartfelt gratitude of those for whom such trifling services were rendered was ample recompense" (67). In fact, the soldiers' appreciation almost undid her, their words, "often more than could be borne" (67), prompting her to disclose a rare moment of emotion as she struggled to remain composed. By way of the rhetoric of the removal of self so that others might speak for her, Holstein accentuated the soldier's gratitude as the embodiment and ultimate test of successful medicine, his "thanks" for her "unskilled hands" amply justifying to her readers the importance of women's work. She upheld the value of her dissent by calling on the judgment of the soldier, thus assuring audience respect.

HOLSTEIN SHOWED two types of linkage in her narrative, the linkage between races, and the linkages between homefront and warfront. Holstein valorized the black soldier, drawing on abolitionist discourse like Powers and other nurses to describe several African American soldiers in camp about whom her readership in Pennsylvania would have been pleased to read. Like most nurse narrators eager to join ranks with the Northern audience at home in conversation about the gains made by abolition, Holstein included admiring descriptions of freedpeople, almost all of them from a measured distance rather than in one-on-one interactions. She contributed heroic portraits of former slaves who expressed "their joy at the sight of the old flag, which *now* meant *freedom* to them" (64).[3] Emphasizing noble, sacrificing black military men, she reported their casualties: "Large numbers of wounded were brought in to-day [July 30th, 1864], principally to the ninth corps and the colored hospital" (82).[4] This reportage almost certainly referred to the soldiers in the 4th Division of the 9th Army Corps in the Battle of the Crater on July 30, 1864, whose enormous sacrifice and valor she noted: "Among the colored troops, *four* out of every five of their officers were either killed or wounded; yet the men behaved bravely" (82).[5]

Holstein heralded the triumph of freedmen serving their country in the procession of a "negro regiment" charged with delivering Southern prisoners of war, among them former slaveholders. A set piece in war literature, Holstein distinguished her scene by utilizing inclusive language in the form of strong pronouns to bolster the differentiation between the "us" and "them." She pointedly grouped the black soldiers with herself and other Northern soldiers and workers, referring to all those parties as "us." The term "them" meant white Southerners: "Eight hundred captured rebels brought in, guarded by a negro regiment—the most humiliating thing to *them* [the Confederates] that could have occurred" (72). Holstein compounded the drama by pointing out the action of "one of our [black] men," who recognized "his former owner, ran up with a pleased look to speak to Massa Charles, but he [Charles] refused to recognize him, and moved on with the crowd" (72). This scene of a black soldier guarding a white prisoner who was formerly his slaveholder focused on an advancing change in American identity whereby the freedman secured the principles of liberty for the country. Observing the black regiment with pride, Holstein showed how cultural structures were being recast, so that a freedman soldier was now "one of our men," policing Southern white prisoners. The entire camp, black and white, hurried to take part in the event, to witness the black troops marching rebels through the camp, to honor these soldiers evidencing their heroism and mastery in the line of duty, and to celebrate the rightful reassignment of power.[6]

In another kind of linkage—that between homefront and warfront—Holstein reminded her audience of the connection between "fronts" that connected women working for Union soldiers. The homefront and warfront linkage endured in Holstein's extended travels, which extended throughout her memoir. The homefront-warfront connection was discussed at some length in other chapters, as in Alcott's play on the word, "war-fare," which coupled domestic and military terms. Holstein melded fronts, too, in effect residing in the crux, which permitted her to impart a discordant picture of domesticity on the move: "our bed was a soldier's couch—the *ground*" (35). At another remove she slept with a "satchel for a pillow" (38), and at yet another, "the deep dust was the only carpet we had" (81). After the battle of Fredericksburg, she cooked at a "camp-stove" that was "very little larger than a lady's band-box," to feed seventy men for several weeks (26). In each of these cases the markers of home interchanged with the exigencies of war.

Perhaps the longest integrated narrative sequence in *Three Years in Field*

Hospitals had to do precisely with showing such vexed combinations of the demarcations of war and home when the army camped by Potomac Creek very near the front. Over the course of several months the troops had settled into a field location for so long they undertook beautification projects, planting flowers and vegetables in order to give the soldiers meaningful work and resulting comfort. Holstein noted in particular that "in front of our tent was a rustic arbor, so complete that any of our country homes would prize it for its beauty" (30). This gardening project transformed the grounds into settings that were "made *apparently* as lasting as though we expected to spend the summer within sight and sound of rebel batteries" (31). Suddenly, on June 13, 1863, while they dined, the order came at a moment's notice to strike camp: all soldiers, upon hearing the signal, jumped to the task of collapsing the facility, and "in *two hours* the seven hundred men were on their way" (31). The most salient detail of this instant removal showed in one worker's precipitous end to his gardening activity: "the gardener was putting the finishing touches to some ornamental rustic work about our tent: *instantly* hammer and hatchet were thrown aside" (31). After the hundreds of soldiers readied themselves, they torched the area: "We sat, quietly watching the flames as they curled and flashed from one arbor to another, encircling in a wall of fire the evergreen screens which had so pleasantly shielded us from heat and dust" (32). What the soldiers couldn't ignite they axed, the destruction the more poignant for being, of necessity, self-inflicted.[7]

In another instance of the uncomfortable conjunction of homefront and warfront, Holstein described a massive explosion that occurred at City Point, Virginia, on August 9, 1864, as she "was occupied in the arbor in front of our tent," perhaps tending plants, when she was "with the first shock stooped to the earth, as though struck upon the head; the tent quivered as though it *must* fall" (85). The seismic blast shook the camp: "There now rose to a great height a dense column of smoke, spreading out at the top in form of an umbrella, and from it fell a shower of death-dealing missiles; it literally *rained* muskets" (85). The surreal scene underscored the violence and incongruity of extended inhabitation of a war zone, where borders could boast arbors and gardens at any moment to give way to an umbrella cloud raining muskets.[8] As her work traversed many margins of war zones, areas that were in flux, she developed the ability to cope with the disorder, an ability that became, for several years, a way of life.[9,10]

IF ANNA MORRIS HOLSTEIN had much to say about travel, dissent, and linkages, she had even more to say about horror and the dead line, which she observed firsthand in four of the most devastating fronts for Civil War casualties: Antietam; Gettysburg; the 1864 campaign of the Army of the Potomac; and Annapolis, Maryland, where the former prisoners from the camp in Andersonville, Georgia were attended. Concerning the first of these, the 1862 Battle of Antietam, Holstein declared, "the name of Antietam is ever associated in my mind with scenes of horror" (11). In describing the battle aftermath she may have referenced for her reader the settings of Antietam associated with the desolation captured in the photography of Alexander Gardner, displayed within weeks of the battle at Mathew Brady's New York studio. Brady's exhibition, called "The Dead of Antietam," depicted the wrenching images of corpses lining a country road that shocked viewers unused to seeing such a display of bodies of the dead: "The photographs gave the public their first look at war—and their *reactions* became news as reporters struggled to describe to the absent nation the simultaneous allure and horror that drew crowds to the viewing" (Stout 158). News of Brady's realistic photos of carnage may have braced Holstein so she could aim a similar lens of steadiness on her own depictions. In fact, perhaps aspiring to Brady's fatalism in her graphic accounts, she began her narrative with the havoc at Antietam.

Holstein found a break with patriotic American war rhetoric that would, in light of her unflinchingly realist outlook, widen throughout the course of the narrative. Witnessing an unending stream of incoming wounded from Antietam, Holstein saw so many bodies that they came to seem to her almost interchangeable: "When a soldier dies, his vacant place upon the floor is soon filled by another; and so the *number* remains the same" (22). Holstein offered a surreal calculus of war injuries, and continued to report countless casualties at the White House on the Pamunkey River, too, where "day and night the interminable trains continued, bringing thousands of wounded men, with the dust and smoke of battle yet upon them" (66). The "interminable trains" began to haunt the narrative: "*Acres* of ground were soon covered with bleeding, mangled men . . . thousands not even shielded from the burning sun" (66). She described also the devastation at Gettysburg, where the Gettysburg soldiers "had stood as a 'living wall' between us and the foe" (40):

> one *great* hillock would be pointed out where *hundreds*, perhaps, had sternly fought and bravely fallen. To persons unfamiliar with such things, as sad a sight as any are the heaps of blood-stained clothing, the shattered muskets, the discarded knapsacks, disabled cannon and caissons, and the innumerable heaps of slain horses which literally cover the hard-fought field. (39–40)

The massive toll on human life at Gettysburg, as at Antietam, was difficult to register, the images harrowing.

Other memoirs did not go into such detail, as one critic asserts of the typical soldier's account, which "doesn't deal much with the horrors of war, tending to focus on the ironic" (Hawk, "Behind the Front Lines"). Perhaps this factor spoke to the incomprehensibly hostile reader review that saw Holstein's memoir as "unhappily marked by a temper more patriotic than generous. The authoress may have been distinguished in works of patriotism and charity, but she can certainly claim no exemption from the narrowness of spirit and pettiness of malice which ill-nature attributes to feminine patriots" (*Littell's* June 29, 1867). In many veterans' memoirs, the soldiers might write of wounds to underscore bravery, but Holstein's narrative documented the war's massive havoc, as Brady's photographs did.[11] Her extensive representations of carnage were also not standard for the nurse narrative, though some—Bucklin in particular—offered detailed descriptions of annihilation. More often, however, nurses would leaven their presentation of suffering with other ameliorating considerations, such as a story of a favorite soldier's recovery.

At times, Holstein's break with patriotic American war rhetoric enlarged into what was almost a counter-rhetoric. She wrote in constant awareness of mortality, the relentless mayhem prompting her grisly but understandable obsession with the edge at which either existence or extinction would take precedence; this was the dead line. Starting by describing the men who were at the edge of death when she was at Antietam, she then addressed a vastly different horror when she witnessed the returning Andersonville prisoners at war's end. Not until that point did she use the phrase "dead line"—a piercing term which is borrowed here for the purposes of *Civil War Nurse Narratives* to convey and understand Holstein's obsession with the line at which life or death obtained. The dead line, a liminal space, engraved the thin fissure between existence and termination. She was not alone in this preoccupation and vigilance, of course, for Elvira Powers, too, mentioned "crossing the line" several times in the same context, as did Whitman after them, in his *Memoranda during the War*, evoking patriotically "the dead line, over which so many brave soldiers pass'd to the freedom of eternity" (Whitman 58).

Holstein's accounts were disturbing in that she did not place the accounts in a framework of freedom or bravery, as for example in the story of a young wife who traveled to see her wounded husband at Antietam. Holstein relayed the wife's discovery that her husband had died and been buried two days before her arrival and, apparently unable to accept his death, she demanded to see his body; as it was exhumed, she "clutched the earth by handfuls" to speed the process, only to find at the bottom of the grave his corpse, and the proof of his decease (13). Holstein captured the bleak emotional details of the graveside scene without adding any mitigating comfort. The fact of the death of a loved one is difficult for any survivor to grasp, but the brutal conditions of the war made acceptance extremely difficult, the sudden finality of death far from home slashing a boundary that admitted no return.[12] Holstein offered other examples of exhumations, as for example when a sister requested that a grave be reopened so that she could "know that it was *indeed* her brother" (17).

Scenes of interments, disinterments, and reinterments demonstrated Holstein's staunch resolve to report wartime mortalities, including the cases of those who strangely appeared not to stay dead, or appeared to arise from the dead, or would seem to hover at the line as if attempting to find a way back from termination. In one case, a man fell in battle, and the funeral sermon was preached over his body on the spot, though later, "when the wounded were gathered up," his comrades discovered him blinded, but alive (49). Indeed, portions of Holstein's memoir would appear to stray almost into gothic literature except that her style was so direct and her medium so solidly nonfiction. But to suggest that such incidents could seem fantastic or macabre does not deny the seriousness of the events of the war; on the contrary, it allots full compass to war experience as perceived by nurses like Holstein, who of course had little recourse to making full sense of such ongoing onslaught while in the midst of it.[13]

Occasionally she drew slightly less horrific scenes, too, with semi-comic tones. For example, she described an incident that almost became a live burial: the body of a soldier was being carried to the grave, when the couch he was resting on was jolted by the bearers, "the man—dead, as they supposed—raised his head and called in a clear voice: 'Boys, what are you doing?'" (41). When they told him, he responded: "'I don't see it, boys; give me a drink of water, and carry me back," adding, as he glanced into the grave and recognized the corpse of an officer, "'I won't be buried by this raw recruit!'" (41–42). Holstein recounted this tale of humor in which the soldier, speaking with Davy Crockett–like audacity, returned to life.[14]

From this point on, though, she almost never alleviated her account with tales in that lighter tone, and continued on with grim documentation. Around mid-narrative, during her description of the 1864 campaign of the Army of the Potomac, Holstein recorded "a train of wounded five miles in length," and added that she didn't know how the estimate came about, but that she could attest that the hospital workers thought the line of casualties "*never* would end" (70). She also reported that her daily life was so crowded with the injured she couldn't walk without taking care not to disturb them: "Nothing before us all the day but wounded; wounded men at every step you take" (76). Perhaps most painful of all, the patients began again to seem replaceable, as they had at Antietam: "The first boat-load [was] sent off to-day, June 20th; but others directly fill their places" (77). In the economy of war, the relief workers had to give efficient, almost assembly-line treatment to the wounded after big battles, and in doing so they lost track of faces and personalities, to risk losing track of humanity altogether.

By the end of *Three Years* Holstein had become even more engrossed in the line between life and death, as the war's escalation dictated the need for nurses to tend to a burgeoning number of casualties. Even the landscape evoked horror: "The dust continues fearfully deep; it is the only thing that moves about *freely*" (80). A troubling sentence for a narrator in an American war describing an American landscape, the statement called into question the country's very reliance on the rudimentary concept of liberty, her emphasis on the word "*freely*" designating dust rather than people as the agent able to move of its own will. Chillingly, Holstein cast doubt upon the nation's fresh form of democratic government by implying it might not survive the conflict. She served notice on an American landscape consigned to the preeminence of nothingness: "Passed, both going and returning, through most fearfully desolate-looking country" (89). Ruined in all directions, both going and returning, destruction and death were inescapable.

In the last and longest chapter, which covered the final year of the war and afterwards, Anna Morris Holstein devoted her attention solely to the soldiers released from Southern prison camps and returning to the Annapolis Barracks. Unlike the men who seemed to "come back" to life in the early parts of the narrative, these last patients seemed to undergo the opposite, as they endured torturous recoveries to survive in a kind of living death. Holstein admitted at this point that she had come up against the limits of representation, that she felt constrained to write about what was "too terrible to be lightly spoken, and too painful in its remembrances to be dwelt upon any longer than is needful for the connected continuance of the narrative" (91). In the above line, she exhibited the discursive dilemma of a writer attempting to articulate the sufferings of prisoners of war, aware on the one hand of the danger of omitting wrenching details and thereby denying the whole truth, and on the other hand of lingering inhumanely on patients' agony. That is to say, over-reporting could surfeit the limits of representation and tip into sensationalism.[15] Poised to navigate this ethical dilemma, Holstein seized upon the self-imposed mandate to report the events in her narrative as she saw them, chronicling with painful clarity the sufferings of some thousands of returning captives.

She often portrayed the returning prisoners as the "living expired," as in the example of one man whose entire face had "an unearthly, smoke-dried parchment look," and who was only seventeen years of age, but looked "at least *forty*" (92). Another, also a skeleton, had lost all his hair except for one tuft, his head and neck "eaten in great holes by vermin" (121). In one arrival of 200 soldiers, the men could not be made to understand that they "*would be* provided for; but clutched with a firm grasp the bones and scraps which they had concealed" (109), and in another group of 460 men, the majority were unable to walk, one-third of them having turned "imbecile" (95). Holstein gave numerous accounts of men with severe mental disabilities, as in the case of the soldier who, when asked his identity, answered with a different name every time (118). She described many instances, too, of what today would be called post-traumatic stress disorder, but then was called "irritable heart." According to Jeff Wheelwright, "Among the [Civil War] amputees, morphine addicts, and war-torn 'insane' were pensioners who had been weakened by 'irritable heart'" (Wheelwright 18), a Civil War condition caused by psychological stress.

As the reports of atrocities at prison camps run by both the Union and Confederate armies surfaced, Americans were left grasping for a way to place Civil War experience within any kind of humane framework. Attempting to express such experience strained the possibilities of discourse, as one returning soldier said: "'We can never tell the half of all we have endured; it would not be credited, if we did'" (Holstein 91). In other words, even if the teller could find the words, the listener would not have the capacity to receive, or even believe it. For a memoirist like Holstein, such a rhetorical standoff challenged her to attempt to discover discursive solutions, despite the fact that they were not always available. In *The Body in Pain*, the landmark study on the suffering and inflicting of pain, Elaine Scarry argues that by its very nature pain resists representation, suggesting the difficulty of both delivering and receiving such an account: "When one hears about another person's physical pain,"

Scarry states, "the events happening within the interior of that person's body may seem to have the remote character of some deep subterranean fact, belonging to an invisible geography that, however portentous, has no reality because it has not yet manifested itself on the surface of the earth" (3).[16]

Grappling with these impasses in representation, Holstein attempted to voice the reality of the afflictions she had witnessed to Americans who had not seen warfare firsthand on such a large, systemic, and familial scale. Nowhere did she challenge the American ethos more than in this last chapter. The closest she came to solving the quandary of voicing events that by their very nature evade or override existing discourse because the reality "has not yet manifested itself on the surface of the earth" was to suggest that lives were lost in the cause of abolition: "The costly offering was asked for, and given, that the nation might be saved, and that distant lands might learn to what refinements of cruelty SLAVERY had educated a people!" (109). Attempting to imbue with meaning the horrifying results of incarceration in the prison camps, Holstein suggested that only abolitionism afforded the possibility of justifying such horrors, and more, that abolition might be able to teach other lands to liberate people and avoid a cataclysm. If the war abolished slavery, then perhaps not all purpose had disintegrated. In this way, she cast a hope that she had not broken entirely with the rhetoric of American patriotism and that war suffering might be eased in the future, if the country could rediscover in emancipation an enduring "liberty for all."

In parts of Holstein's account, however, she simply could not procure meaning for the agony prisoners had undergone, and one final incident served to show the line at which, for her, ethical import lingered then disintegrated altogether. Holstein related a story of the abhorrent treatment of two Union prisoners of war who approached the "'dead line'" of Andersonville prison camp. The dead line, which indicated the camp's boundary inside the boundary, constituted "a crude one-rail fence [which] ran parallel to the interior wall of the stockade, creating a fifteen-foot buffer zone between the prisoners and the wall" (Walker 110). Both Southern and Northern prison camps used the dead line as a demarcation for the line beyond which a prisoner could not move without the risk of a guard

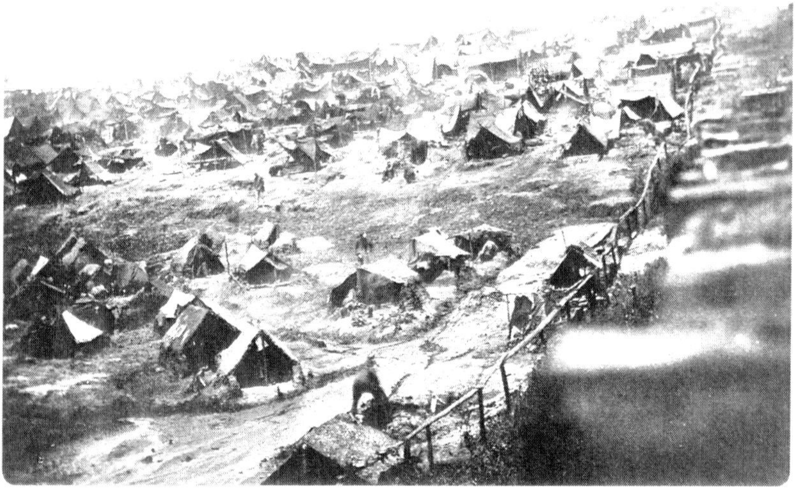

Andersonville, Georgia, 1864, with southwest view of stockade showing the dead line
Courtesy of the Library of Congress

opening fire. The dead line formed "perhaps the greatest symbol of violence at Andersonville" (Walker 110), and Holstein used the term to show gross inhumanity. In the story of the two prisoners, the men walked to find water near the line and were tempted to move closer to the stream by a tower guard who threw a piece of bread down near one man: "eagerly the hand was outstretched to grasp it, the fingers up to the 'line,' when, in an instant, his brains were scattered upon the cup and bread he held!" (122). Holstein emphasized the premeditated malignity of the guard who used a feint of kindness to commit an act of brutality. The dead line, an actual prison border, suggested for the purposes of Holstein's narrative the border across which human actions should not be admissible, across which language can hardly manage to match word to deed.

No wonder Holstein wrote in her introduction that "the events of the war are 'graven as with an iron pen' upon my memory" (v). She admitted such a crushing several-week period of increases in mortalities that her narrative line sputtered: "my notes were too hurried and unsatisfactory for reference; they merely repeat that one and another has passed 'to the land of rest'" (42). At the end, war service must have undone her to some extent, at least for a while, given that she wrapped up her book with two paragraphs not characterized by statements of unmitigated fact, but by platitudes that fell altogether flat of narrative denouement, in no way contextualizing the ravages she had witnessed.[17] Offering a gruesome critique of the project of war suffering, she only rarely alleviated that critique by voicing the hope that abolition could help the nation come to terms. Holstein posed an interrogation of suffering that by default admitted the impossibility of gaining compass on the subject of death, ultimately refusing to profess that compensation existed for such massive pain, such slaughter, and the existence of the dead line.

Each race saw the other . . . (367)

CHAPTER SIX

Sophronia Bucklin's *In Hospital and Camp*

Rank-and-File Nursing

In the several pages of recommendations that preceded Sophronia Bucklin's narrative proper, surgeon after surgeon attested to Bucklin's excellence as a nurse, bestowing praise with such often-repeated words as "faithful," "indefatigable," and "industrious." Bucklin would have had to possess these traits even to begin to find a way to join the war effort, given that she would have been disqualified for being under thirty-five years of age, which was seen as "altogether too young for a nurse" (Bucklin 60). Further, the government stipulated that she "must be of strong health—not subject to chronic diseases, nor liable to sudden illnesses," and that she "must present certificates of qualification and good character" (39). In addition, according to Bucklin, the general populace had a predisposition to rebuff female nurses in general: "'It is no place for women,' was the cry on every hand" (35)[1] Bucklin thus felt fortunate to happen on a connection while working at the Orphan Asylum in

Auburn, New York, to secure a meeting with the Board of Managers for the Soldiers Aid Society of Auburn, and to be signed on by Dorothea Dix to work for the Army of the Potomac from September 1862 and throughout the war.

Traveling to a new location was full of challenges for nurses, as we have seen, and Bucklin's experience was no exception. She noted her entry into Washington, DC, which she characterized as dark, "as though the smoke from a thousand grim throated furnaces had settled upon its walls, and thousands of soldiers had shook there the dust from their feet, brought from every State in the Union" (43). Bucklin went to Washington to attend to American soldiers and found herself vitally interested in finding justice for the rank-and-file soldier, including fair treatment for patients, due respect for those of different social classes, and, in the end, fair treatment for people both black and white. Inscribing a rhetoric of patriotism and women's rights, she created a tie with her reader, delivering this statement as her motivation for serving: "The same patriotism which took the young and brave from the workshop and plow, from counting-rooms, and college halls . . . lent also to our [female] hearts its thrilling measure, and sent us out to do and dare . . ." (33). The three main segments of this chapter follow Bucklin's actions of dissent, her camaraderie with the working-class soldier, and her growing support for the social rights of freedpeople as she worked alongside and supervised black workers and soldiers.

SOPHRONIA BUCKLIN dissented against officials whose neglectful actions affected the well-being of her patients. Of the seven nurse narrators studied in this book, Bucklin devised the most resourceful means of voicing disaffection within the hospital institution. Schultz comments that Bucklin had the "spirit of rebellion" (137), and "portrayed herself as a righteous commando" (240) and indeed, she filled *In Hospital and Camp* with the tales of a woman bent on confronting officials she saw as exploitative. Most often female nurses were disposed to laud rather than criticize physicians, singling out those who treated soldiers with kindness; Elvira Powers, for instance, praised a doctor who refused oys-

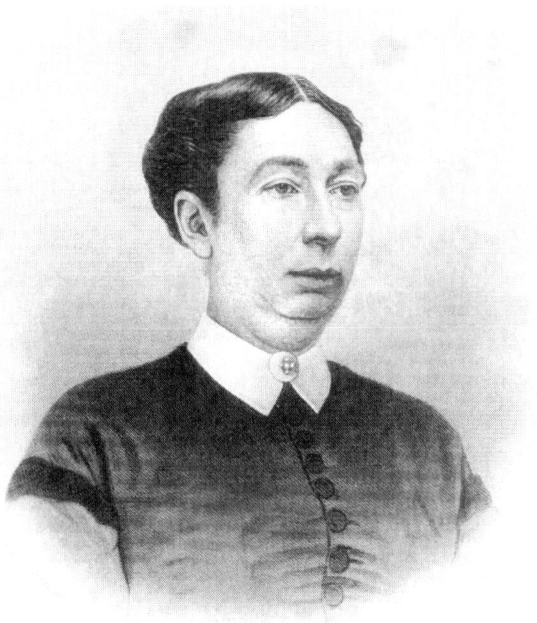

Sophronia Bucklin

Sophronia Bucklin, *In Hospital and Camp*, 1869

ters at his dinner table because the soldiers had no such fare at theirs (53). Bucklin, too, mentioned cases in which surgeons and other officials worked together to promote the health and comfort of the wounded and sick, but when officials were self-serving, she used her narrative to speak out. In her handwritten manuscript of *In Hospital and Camp*, Bucklin offered an instructive example of how she fueled her righteous anger when confronting physicians guilty of graft and cruelty. In the manuscript, she altered the phrase "narrow sould [*sic*] men" (Bucklin Papers, Folder 21) by crossing out the word "men" and adding "selfish men," so that the phrase appeared in the final publication as "narrow-souled, selfish men" (175).[2] Apparently she wasn't content with denouncing incompetent doctors only in the Christian rhetoric of the soul but also wanted invective that denounced their characters on the basis of worldly failings, and so added the secular word "selfish" to drive home her point.

On the first page of *In Hospital and Camp* Bucklin defended her acts of dissent, leaving no doubt as to the two forms of rhetoric on which she relied. First, her core discourse was undergirded by principles of patriotism—or more specifically, a patriotic civil disobedience with an elegant pedigree: the Declaration of Independence. Second, her go-to rhetoric was that of women's rights. Bucklin devised an astute way to ally the two forms of discourse, as we can see in the book's first sentence, in which Bucklin justified dissent by alluding to the Declaration. She used its precise voicing to provide a stepping-off place for her own writing:

> When, in the complexity of national affairs, it became necessary for armed men to assemble in multitudes, to become exposed to the hardships and privations of camps and the deadly peril of battle fields, there arose the same necessity for woman to lend her helping hand to bind up the wounds of the shattered soldier, and smooth the hard pillow of the dying hero. (33)

Bucklin mirrored the outlook of much of the Northern populace by stating that the nation faced a crisis at least equal to that of the Revolutionary War, but notably, she designated the actions of women as parallel in importance to those of men. Concerned with the material world, with palpable exigencies, and with gender, she established the crucial need for the actions of men *and* women, each responding out of "the same necessity"; this phrase established the cornerstone for her argument that women owned the right to serve as nurses and to speak out as nurses.

For comparison, here is the first sentence of the Declaration of Independence itself:

> When in the Course of human events, it becomes necessary for one people to dissolve the political bands which have connected them with another, and to assume, among the Powers of the earth, the separate and equal station to which the Laws of Nature and of Nature's God entitle them, a decent respect to the opinions of mankind requires that they should declare the causes which impel them to the separation. (Beschloss 11)

Using the logic of a conditional statement, the Declaration states that when historical circumstances reach a boiling point, to the extent that it becomes incumbent on one set of people to "dissolve" their connections with another and to set up a separate "station" to which they are entitled by nature and God, then they should in all decency express the reasons why. Needless to say, Thomas Jefferson and the intrepid Sophronia Bucklin spoke from different circumstances and to more or less different purposes. Whereas the Declaration depended on comprehensive abstractions, such as "the Powers of the earth," "the Laws of Nature and of Nature's God," and "the opinions of mankind," Bucklin's sallied forth with cold, hard details, such as "the hardships and privations of camp," "the wounds of the shattered soldier," and "the hard pillow of the dying hero."

Yet another document, however, parallels Bucklin's opening salvo, one penned in the time frame between the Declaration of 1776 and Bucklin's personal declaration of 1869. This document, written in 1848, originated at the Woman's Rights Convention at Seneca Falls:

> When, in the course of human events, it becomes necessary for one portion of the family of man to assume among the people of the earth a position different from that which they have hitherto occupied . . . [then] they [women] should declare the causes that impel them to such a course. (Stanton, *History* 70).

The Seneca Falls document echoed the first sentence of the original Declaration very closely, almost word for word, suggesting female independence in the right to "Life, Liberty and the pursuit of happiness"; women had a radical obligation to undertake action "whenever a government becomes destructive of these ends" by insisting on "a new government" (70). Bucklin's affirmation of the woman nurse's prerogatives echoed both the 1776 and 1848 declarations, relying on both patriotic rhetoric and women's rights rhetoric to legitimate the woman nurse's right to take action in the cause of her country.[3] From the vantage of such perspicacious documents, Bucklin rallied toward greater justice, assuming the authority to act on behalf of patients, action which later carried over to dissent.

Bucklin may have seen more types of official neglect and abuse than other nurses, given that she was shuffled to many different wards and camps in the course of her service. Discharged and reinstated several times, she distinguished herself both positively and negatively to a number of authorities, undertaking both loyal service and noteworthy dissent in various jobs. Because of varying appointments over years' worth of service, she had ample time to develop and alter strategies as she became more nimble at expressing disagreement. As in Powers's case, the word "dissent" covered Bucklin's response to a wide scope of workplace conflicts, including tactics used to manage disagreement. Her tactics covered four basic strategies: interpretation, appeal, noncompliance, and confrontation. The first two—interpretation and appeal—she used to dispel workplace conflict, and the second two—noncompliance and confrontation—to dispute authority. Each strategy spoke to a woman's right to hold a job in the service of her country, and all were devised to create a bond with the women readers of Bucklin's narrative.

The first of the four strategies, interpretation, was employed to counter rules Bucklin found arbitrary and senseless while she kept the appearance of following them; by interpreting regulations, she could avoid disturbance while effecting good for the patient. Allied to the rhetorical tactics of indirection and deflection, interpretation was used to waylay conflict but also went one step further, into action. Early on in the narrative, Bucklin developed interpretation so she could serve soldiers the particular food and drink they wanted, as when she and the other nurses at Judiciary Square Hospital bypassed obstructionist orders to provide harmless, "little comforts" to soldiers craving particular refreshments. She and her female coworkers "smuggled" tea to the patients, a substance forbidden by the rules, by way of "slipping a basin of water into the stove in the ward" and "dropping the tea into it when boiling," after which they took the basin to their quarters and returned carrying "it thence in a bowl, having all the appearance of official ordering" (59). By essentially repackaging the tea in the official-looking bowls, and feigning obedience to the letter of the law, they initiated the means to offer patients a comforting, perhaps restorative drink. Such use of rule interpretation avoided ruffling feathers and evaded the danger of punishment in the face of what might otherwise have ended in contretemps. This early example of dissent was additionally remarkable because the women bent the rule together, in solidarity.

With the tea episode Bucklin hinted at but didn't embrace defiance, stating her position as such: "Surgeons and officers were very kind to us, but they gave stringent orders which we were sometimes almost willing to disobey" (59). Offering a caveat to the option of disobedience by using the qualifiers "sometimes" and "almost," Bucklin described with trenchant irony the nurses' willingness to interpret but not altogether to contravene the rules. As Bucklin's narrative progressed, though, her qualifiers became less pronounced and she accelerated beyond the "almost" into willingness to disobey. Anticipating future actions, she suggested that, "the red tape, as the soldiers termed it, required too much official ceremony in the untying—we would rather break the string, and in serving the wounded hurriedly throw away the pieces" (59).

Soon after the tea incident, disagreements with authorities flared into bigger disputes, requiring her to move from interpretation to the more open tactic of appeal, which she applied especially in a series of power struggles pertaining to her right to cook for patients. Starting at Point Lookout Hospital, Maryland, she developed a kind of cookstove dissent over control of the key to the food cupboard, and ended with an out-and-out battle over a cookstove at City Point Hospital, Virginia. Discord arose from a string of kitchen altercations, often spurred by her suspicion that the ward master, or other officials, were withholding needed nourishment and comforts from patients, and sometimes spurred by the conjecture that the reason was graft: "*Some one* was living on the rations of these poor men, who were suffering and starving for the want of them" (93).[4]

The first kitchen discord began when Bucklin was inadvertently caught in a power struggle between the ward surgeon and the steward, the first of whom gave her the key to the cupboard and the second of whom reprimanded her for being in possession of that same key, thereby having "usurped his position" (96). The steward confronted her during rounds, charged her with the infraction of possessing the key, and relieved her of duty. In response, she appealed immediately to the hospital matron, who managed to set up a meeting whereby Bucklin could explain the case to the surgeon in charge. Happening to be summoned as she stood in the kitchen making gingerbread dough, she talked to the surgeon in charge with her "doughy hands and sleeves pinned up" (98), and as a result of their conversation, he countermanded her discharge. Astonishingly, later the same day, Bucklin was served her "*second* relief papers," thus impelled again to contact the matron, the two women running to the wharf to waylay the same surgeon in charge so that he could countermand the order a second time, which he did. Afterward, though, the unscrupulous steward seemed to concoct punitive rules for the pleasure of commanding Bucklin; for instance, he told her she must desist from cooking eggs on the stove, despite the fact that a physician consulting with her had expressly ordered eggs for a particular patient. She discussed the steward's order with the physician, who counseled her to cook not *on* the stove but *in* it: "'Jam everything you want to cook *into* the stove, there isn't an order against that'" (100). She used the physician's useful loophole.

Her cooking exploits continued when later on, in her service at City Point Hospital, Bucklin circumvented what seemed to her nonsensical orders concerning the use of another cookstove; indeed, one interchange reached the point of absurdity, wherein she was "interrogated" concerning her "extra cooking again" (323). The charge that she had committed the crime of extra cooking was questionable, if not ludicrous, given that her objective was to make nutritious, appealing food for patients. At another location, "Wolf-Street Hospital" in Alexandria, Virginia, Bucklin was delivered dismissal papers, then reinstated by Superintendent Dix, then dismissed again. Reminiscent of Powers's experience, Bucklin's experience included not being told the nature of her "crime," and being astonished at the news. Unable to imagine what had prompted her sudden termination, Bucklin asserted that she had "not the slightest idea of the charges brought against me" (132). The dismissal turned out, again, to be for the apparent crime of extra cooking: she had awakened before hours to make biscuits for breakfast, and the biscuits had not been officially sanctioned.

At City Point Hospital, Bucklin once again was caught between command styles, this time between the efficient Dr. Hammond and the reportedly incompetent Dr. Frederick Burmeister, the latter of whom both preceded and succeeded Dr. Hammond as the surgeon in charge. Clearly, soldiers as well as nurses were at times starving or nearly so at City Point under Burmeister, under whose direction meals consisted at times of

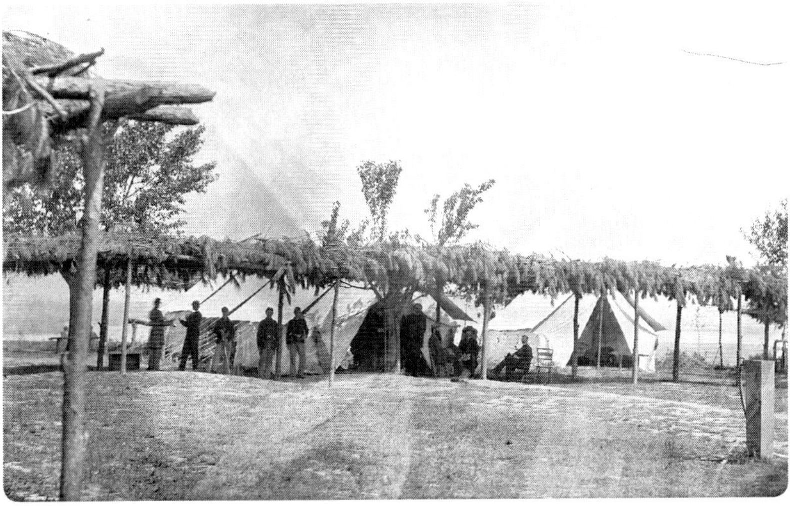

Tents of the General Hospital at City Point, Virginia

Courtesy of the Library of Congress

"wormy, mouldy 'hard tack,'" burned cornstarch thrown in a tub and "allowed to stand until it had a green mould over the surface," and soup of the "poorest quality" with only bits of dried bread in it (290). Bucklin didn't know if the conditions arose from the surgeon-in-charge's "neglect or want of executive ability"—but in any case, "matters grew worse" (291). When Hammond took over City Point, the change in leadership improved conditions overnight, and when Bucklin forthrightly asked him for a cook stove, he followed through directly, procuring her the means to make cakes, pies, biscuits, and other food for the patients. Though she incurred the jealousy of some of the other nurses who apparently lacked the energy or desire to make baked goods for their patients, Bucklin retained Hammond's support and on his advice she continued her labors "in silence" (304).

Burmeister succeeded Hammond, however, to become surgeon-in-charge again, and at this point Burmeister pushed Bucklin to act in noncompliance. Burmeister "boarded" (322) with one of the nurses, who complained to him of Bucklin, and perhaps as a consequence he decided to requisition the cookstove, leaving her, no doubt, furious. Bucklin immediately went into action, applying to the Christian Commission for a "larger and better" stove (322), and when it arrived, Burmeister requisitioned that one, too. Exasperated but undeterred Bucklin, in a breathtaking act of agitation, traveled to Washington "without Dr. Burmeister's knowledge" (323) to buy a stove with her own money and have it shipped back to City Point. In this riposte, Burmeister apparently judged her act of noncompliance to be that of insubordination, for on learning of the transgression he sent out a search party, as she reported: "the corporal and guard had been out all day in search of me" (330). Aware of the potential punishment for her behavior, Bucklin resolutely claimed, "I did not fear the guard-house," because "brave soldiers had been innocently thrust into it" (330). She braced herself with the logic that guiltless troops had been wrongfully punished in this way, so she could withstand it, too; allying herself with the rank-and-file men, she was prepared for the same consequences.

Some of Bucklin's deliberations defined the cusp at which resistance became conscionable and even necessary in order to be a responsible American, as defined in the Declaration, which scripted disobedience as part-and-parcel of civic commitment.[5] Such considerations had operated at the forefront of abolitionist deliberations for years, especially when the 1850 Fugitive Slave Act tipped the scales of protest, making it necessary for abolitionists to grapple with the question of performing the illegal act of abetting or harboring a fugitive slave. Bucklin may have reasoned that if an abolitionist needed sometimes to act judiciously on the nether side of the law, so did she when she flouted Burmeister's expectations about the cookstove. She inflamed his wrath and risked incarceration, knowing that the deck was stacked against errant female nurses: "Many surgeons, at this date of the war, were determined, by a systematic course of ill-treatment toward women nurses, to drive them from the service" (124). Given her reliance on declarations of Americans' and women's independence, it is likely that her breaches of protocol were conscious and considered.

Throughout these episodes Bucklin plied various modes of dissent —interpretation, appeal, and noncompliance—but stopped short of the most extreme mode of outright confrontation. But that was soon to come. She finally transferred to Point of Rocks, Maryland, but during her new assignment returned to City Point to recoup her clothing, and found that her stove had arrived. Due to the mistake of a "half-drunken clerk," however, it had been addressed to Superintendent Dix instead of Bucklin. She tried to reason with the clerk, asking him to send it to her instead of Dix, arguing that her clothes were stored in the boiler of the stove, but he refused. Finally, Bucklin intimidated a surgeon by stating that she would turn the matter over to the provost marshal and, surprisingly, the surgeon capitulated, stipulating minor conditions but finally handing over her "long coveted stove" (336). With this final installment in the chronicle of the cookstove, Bucklin demonstrated that she could, at least in this instance, use confrontation to pressure an authority with an ultimatum and get what she wanted.[6]

Finally, Bucklin recorded an altogether different struggle over abuse of power, which occurred in the form of sexual harassment. Other nurse narrators may have omitted the issue because it did not speak to patients' rights, a cause they felt relatively comfortable raising in the name of patriotism and justice; by contrast, they would have hesitated to raise an issue that had to do with women's rights, for fear of the moral stigma or shame it would place on them. Bucklin, undeterred, told in her narrative the story of the surgeon in charge at Camp Stoneman, Washington, DC, who sexually mistreated a woman, a Mrs. Bolier, who arrived to nurse her dying husband. Over the course of time this surgeon in charge made "infamous proposals" and "a fiendish spirit tempted the surgeon in charge to insult" (240) the woman. Mrs. Bolier rejected these "advances," and as a result the surgeon eventually forbade the woman to enter the ward, causing her great distress. Eventually his harassment left her no recourse other than to leave the hospital. She did so with the assistance of Bucklin, who accompanied her on the first leg of her stagecoach journey home.

After this episode, Bucklin returned to camp and was confronted by the surgeon, livid at her "alleged disobedience" saying, "'If you were a man I would put you in the guard-house'" (241). To this, Bucklin responded with outright aggression: "I replied that he could do so as it was, if he saw fit, but I rather thought he would stand in some danger of losing his other eye (he had lost one), for I had some friends at Camp Stoneman yet—friends, who were well aware of the disgraceful proceedings which had lately been enacted, and who were eager for the opportunity this would afford" (241). Bucklin drew upon the shared values of a group—her friends at Camp Stoneman—to buttress her opprobrium of the "disgraceful proceedings." Combative, she threatened the perpetrator with the loss of his eye, verbally attacking the spot of his greatest vulnerability while punishing the gaze of the eye with which had attempted to control a victim.

Bucklin knew "the tiger was roused in the man—the brute passions were in the ascendant," and after the confrontation chose to report to Superintendent Dix for another assignment rather than continue at that institution. Schultz states that, "by communicating with Dix's office instead of the surgeon's superiors, Bucklin succeeded in having him fired, obtaining a transfer for herself and the other women employed" (138–39); in the end, she probably accomplished less by confrontation than by the ultimate appeal to Superintendent Dix.[7] The episode, which culminated in the surgeon's incarceration in the Old Capital Prison, saw him "court-martialed, his pay withheld, and himself disgraced and dismissed from the service" (244). It was a marked punishment for a surgeon whose demise could be chalked up at least partly to the otherwise institutionally powerless Bucklin, who crossed the gender boundaries of prescriptive female behavior.[8]

BUCKLIN'S PARTICULAR STRIPE of rank-and-file entailed of necessity a well-developed respect for the working class. Like many other women nurses, she predicated the value of her contribution to the war effort precisely upon the soldier's appreciation of her work:

> Officers now and then threw out hints that women were a nuisance in war. We cared little. . . . We knew that many a poor wounded fellow blessed in his heart the women. . . . No man of generous heart wished women shut out from the doors of either field or city hospitals. (70–71).

In a deft move, Bucklin differentiated the plural "officers" from the singular "poor wounded fellow," employing the faceless plural to contrast

with the more approachable "fellow." She coded this individual as the more gentlemanly of the two because he had a "generous heart," thus introducing generosity as the distinguishing component of a man's integrity. She contrasted the private with some of the scoundrel officers, whom she characterized as cruel: "It was only the ruffians who feared the just censure of compassionate women" (71).

Bucklin enlarged on the theme of the soldier's grateful acknowledgment of nurses, recalling a patient who said that it "'*did* do the men *so much good*, to have a woman come, if she didn't say more 'n one word, it revived 'em so'." The working-class soldier praised the female nurse, and the female nurse cared "much more for their [the patients'] approval" than for anything else (172). The common soldier's report was the only recognition a nurse like Sophronia Bucklin would need or want—except for his recovery from wounds or illness, an even more gratifying encomium.

In one instance of the camaraderie between nurse and patient, a "beautiful," dying boy reported to Bucklin, intriguingly, that he had dreamed of her. "During his wild flights in his delirium," Bucklin wrote, "he fancied that they had come to take me to the guard-house, for having cared too much for his comfort" (107). In effect, he showed that he understood the risks she took in dissenting, unconsciously registering that some of her actions in advocacy were the same for which officials might chastise or potentially incarcerate her. The logic of his dream disclosed parallels between nurse compassion and nurse subversion, and his dream amplified the convergence of causes for common soldier and nurse, united by their relative powerlessness but also by their mutual appreciation.

The affinity was conscious too, of course, as Bucklin, Dunlap, Wheelock, and others stated adamantly in their memoirs, prioritizing the needs of the rank-and-file soldier as their democratic imperative. Such nurses used the strategy of camaraderie with a soldier as they did the maternal bond—to strengthen the writer–reader connection. Nurses amplified the personalities of individual patients so as to humanize their work to their readers, thus dramatizing the solidarity between nurses and soldiers who served and sacrificed for the Union cause. Sizer notes that "rather than adopting a professional model of hospital decorum and treating wounded and sick soldiers as nameless patients, nurses sought to retain a sense of the soldier's individual pain" (209). The nurse foregrounded the activities of the less advantaged soldier rather than those of the ranking official, and so personalized him, using a quietly subversive rhetoric interlocking the causes of working-class man with woman nurse. Despite the fact that Bucklin suggested female relief workers did not want or need to claim "the meed of high-sounding praise; we ask not crowns of laurel for our brows" (34), she did record the hearty praise of the ordinary soldier.

When Bucklin first arrived in Washington, tired and hungry, with no "civilized convenience" to offer relief, she began to see herself not only as commensurate with the private but as his cohort, as she was to some extent living the same military life: "A dim sense of what was before me struck upon my understanding, and I began to realize that a soldier's life was anything but pastime" (43). In the introduction to *In Hospital and Camp*, a writer identified as "S. L. C." went further, describing an exact equivalence between female nurse and military man, wherein "for nearly three long years she [Bucklin] led the life of an actual soldier" (21). Bucklin argued class affinity and urged humane treatment for those who were devoted to service: "Nurses and soldiers were supposed, by many of the officers, to be mere machines, incapable of thought, and unworthy of any attention beyond requiring them to be obedient, without questioning whenever their rights were infringed upon" (296). By showing in her account the very human aspects of the "boys," Bucklin blasted the notion that they—soldiers and nurses both—were machines, thus yoking the nurse's history and fortune with that of the private.[9]

Food played an important part in these class struggles, not surprisingly, given that the preparation of food had clarified Bucklin's need to dissent; its distribution further clarified her sense of connection with privates. In contrast to the officers who enjoyed the best of meals, the rank-and-file soldiers and nurses were at times unfairly apportioned food, left to eat "codfish boiled in clear water—hunger being the only sauce" (121), along with what, "aided by a strong imagination," passed for coffee (122). The meager rations left her so weak near the end of one assignment that she "found it necessary to cling to the banisters to assist in ascending the stairs" (122). Bucklin's depiction of this disparity demonstrated a kind of patriotic unity of female nurse with common soldier, each finding solidarity through their common privations.

With such a defense she could suggest fair pay to women nurses—a tricky subject in the mid-nineteenth century, for in the public's mind, the subject was often entangled with suspicion about the nurse's character; many considered a woman's request for an increase in pay as a blemish on a her integrity. A female nurse who asked for compensation might have ulterior motives, as if only those who could afford to do charitable work had good intentions. While some privileged-class nurses could afford to donate labor to the Union effort, others, such as Bucklin, could not, and needed to challenge public perceptions and militate for fair pay. Specifically, Bucklin stated that she earned "forty cents a day and soldier's rations" (70), or, as reported in the introduction, "twelve dollars a month" (22).[10] Bucklin not only made the case, as did other nurses, that the need for wages in no way diminished their patriotism or character, but also argued for parity of payment among nurses within the ranks. In a conversation with Superintendent Dix, Bucklin said she "had not sought or expected ease in coming out to the army," yet she could not understand why women who worked in "post hospitals"—that is, field and camp facilities with rough lodgings and other discomforts and privations—were not paid as well as in women in "general hospitals" (198–99). She understood labor in terms of work difficulty and considered it only fair that the nurse in the field receive the same compensation as the nurse in the urban setting; she wanted not greater, but equal pay.

Bucklin paid attention to matters such as payroll, and as letters from her sister, Almira Chase, reveal, finances proved a constant concern. Elizabeth Leonard's investigation of the letters shows that "from a practical standpoint, Bucklin had to confront the issue of money" (*Yankee* 25). In reading Bucklin's family's letters, one can see that the family needed continually to track their resources and that their interconnections were indexed to some extent according to their economic exigencies; for instance, on September 26, 1862, Chase penned a two-page letter to Bucklin, a good third of which had to do with family finances. Chase tallied her house rent of "one dollar and a quarter a month," her relief money of "5 dollars a month," and the holdings of her soldier son, Charlie, 100 dollars (because an elderly Chase relative had bequeathed "the boys 100 dollars apeace [*sic*]"). Assessing the family's assets, Chase wrote that "Charlie has money" and that "with his bounty money he is going to buy us a house and lot when he comes home if he lives . . . ." These last three words evidenced a stark realism that recalled some of Bucklin's own abrupt language; being direct was apparently part of the Bucklin legacy.

The sisters moved on from the subject of money to the care of family members as more or less inextricable topics. Part of Chase's object in writing seemed to be that she wanted Bucklin to look out for Charlie who had been wounded, shuffled about to different hospitals, discharged, and finally sent home, but now seemed, to his mother's chagrin, anxious to return to duty. Chase may have hoped that her sister could intervene and confessed to her in November 1862 that she wished Charlie would not "be exposed at [*sic*] being out at night on guard or any kind of duty and that he would not have to go in battle, I thought perhaps there might be something he could get into that you would know of" (Papers, Folder 1).

Apparently Bucklin was able to procure a job for her nephew at Point Lookout, as evidenced by Chase's subsequent letter, directed to that location on February 7, addressed to both Sophronia and Charlie. Still deeply concerned with money, Chase urged Bucklin to "let me know some items of what you are appointed to do and tell me how much wages you get a month."[11] Half of the jointly addressed letter was directed to Charlie, almost all of which had to do with family finances, such as the cost of properties in the area and even the selling of his guitar, which fetched "four dollars and fifty cents" (Folder 1). This family pooled their resources, looked out for each other's employment, and watched their pennies.

When Frank Moore put together his collection, *Women of the War; Their Heroism and Self-Sacrifice*, he may have excluded both Powers and Bucklin because they were seen as "troublemakers," Sizer states (208), which was altogether possible, considering the instances of dissent that each woman recorded. Schultz suggests, however, that "it is just as likely that negotiations over money soured Moore, whose middle-class values made him mistrust women seeking pay" (311). If Bucklin had requested remuneration from Moore, he may have jettisoned her contribution because he doubted her integrity, perceiving impropriety in a request that attached payment to authorship.

S. L. C.'s introduction to *In Hospital and Camp* stated the situation even more emphatically: "Who says, because they were paid, the sacrifice which they laid on their country's smoking altar was not a voluntary blood-offering? Who says, because they were furnished subsistence, and were clad, that they died not to save the glorious Union . . . ?" (22–23).[12] S. L. C. used sharp rhetoric to argue that the accomplishments of nurses who risked their lives for the union deserved compensation. As Leonard comments, the "fervor of S. L. C.'s challenge testified to the presence of strong popular sentiment against middle-class women as wage earners" (*Yankee* 27). Sizer assessed the force of S. L. C.'s introduction by considering it next to Bucklin's narrative proper, noting that the introduction's tone "is perhaps more caustic than the text itself" (214). Insisting that soldiers and nurses both deserve encomiums, S. L. C. yoked their contributions, writing that "when the claims of the common soldier have been more fully considered, then will these noble women, who saved thousands of common soldiers to fight again for freedom, find *their* names also inscribed on the long Roll of Honor" (31). In the last sentence of her introduction, S. L. C. charged Bucklin's readership with the task of fair and critical reading, handing over to "a discriminating public this record of the HOSPITAL AND CAMP" (32).

Bucklin herself addressed class issues, though mostly under the auspices of solidarity between nurse and soldier rather than on her own behalf. While she seldom mentioned money concerns, she must have thought about them frequently, given the circumstances of the family finances set forth by Almira Chase. Bucklin eked out a living during the war and in the years afterward, as her papers show: a petition recommending her to the Women's Relief Corps was signed by "the members of the Sydney Post, No. 41, Grand Army of the Republic," from Ithaca, New York, all of whom knew and trusted her to be "worthy of any assistance that may be bestowed on her" (Folder 7). Bucklin also found ways to augment her income, promoting her book with an eye toward sales, even sending a copy of it, during the year of its publication, to the Executive

Mansion in Washington, DC, a fact verified by a record of its receipt, in which a secretary addressed and informed her that "the President requests" the receipt of her book copy be acknowledged (Folder 8). Bucklin may have hoped he would read her work and recommend it to others.

A letter from John E. Potter, the publisher of *In Hospital and Camp*, indicated that Bucklin was to some degree involved personally in the vending of her book, which saw "private printing" (Leonard 161). John Potter responded in detail to a letter from Bucklin asking for "1000 copies," probably so that she could make sales to potential buyers in her area. Apparently concerned about how much she could pay up-front for the copies, Potter warned her that "we should not like any long credits about it" (Folder 8). Even decades later, Bucklin continued to seek support, applying for a pension in 1892, which she was granted in the same year in the amount of "$12" (Conklin 337). Her need continued into her last years, when she turned again to the work of nursing. The City Hospital of Ithaca responded to an inquiry Bucklin sent on January 13, 1901, stating that the hospital "does not graduate nurses but does at times employ probationers" (Folder 8). Bucklin may have been apprehensive about securing a source of income as late as 1901, when she was in her seventies. She died in Ithaca in 1902.

THE THIRD WAY THAT Bucklin demonstrated rank-and-file nursing showed in her interracial interactions, which evolved markedly throughout the memoir. Bucklin did not evince dyed-in-the-wool abolitionist rhetoric as did Alcott, Woolsey, and Powers, but she was nonetheless sympathetic to the antislavery cause. Like other nurse narrators, she engaged in behavior that indicated she was not fully aware of her assumption of white privilege. Bucklin's narrative admitted a window onto her race interactions while also portraying the resistant responses of bondswomen to her presumptive entitlement. Over her years of service, Bucklin underwent a partial change in her outlook concerning race issues whereby she gained mindfulness of her preemptive interchanges.

When she first worked in the fall of 1862 at Thirteenth Street Hospital in Washington, DC, Bucklin witnessed a laundry operation in disarray, with over 500 pieces of sheets, bandages, and garments in various states of mildew and rot, wet with scum and lying in the dirt. Given charge of this laundry operation, Bucklin found that "seven contraband women were still toiling among this condition of things" (68), and she proceeded to divvy up the tasks of washing, ironing, preparing the fires and kettles, fetching water, and folding. Her perception was that the women were "illy [*sic*] inclined to be taught, and somewhat morose about it, but soon recovered their equanimity of spirits" (69). By indicting the women as "morose" and disinclined "to be taught," Bucklin showed an inability to perceive that she was positioned in a racially structured circumstance in which her white perspective coded black women as unteachable. In Chapter 1, Frankenberg's formulations of the three markers of white assumption of privilege were presented: first, "a location of structural advantage" of whiteness; second, a "standpoint or overview of whiteness"; and third, an assumption that these cultural practices are "unmarked and unnamed" (*White Women* 1). Importantly, Frankenberg revised the third formulation to reflect the reality that whiteness "*seems* to be unmarked, but it is in fact rarely so" ("The Critical Study of Whiteness" 116). This third formulation is key, because those *not* in a position of whiteness are most often expressly attuned to such coding and aware of it as a subjugating or intruding condition of their lives.[13] Bucklin came to discern exactly this: that any oppressed people "read" their oppressors as a necessary skill of self-preservation, critically aware that the practices of white entitlement are hardly unmarked, as they perforce shape daily interactions.

One of the crucial understandings of *In Hospital and Camp* rests with the seemingly unmarked nature of Bucklin's white positioning that, albeit unconsciously *to her* (at least at the beginning of her interactions), was anything but uncoded for the enslaved women she supervised. Bucklin disclosed the complicated patterns of white privilege that lacks self-comprehension when she showed herself, almost as case study, to hold two competing outlooks. For example, Bucklin asserted that the women in the laundry were "unused to work where order was to be observed —just loosed from the bonds of slavery, it mattered little to the naturally indolent dispositions of the washerwomen" (69). Bucklin inconsistently attributed both extrinsic and intrinsic causes to the women's behaviors; that is, when she stated that the women were not used to working in an orderly fashion, she acknowledged that the oppressive circumstances of slavery had conditioned their behavior, but when she referred to the women as "naturally" indolent, she ascribed their behavior as innate—instead of also conditioned by slavery[14] As Susan M. Ryan observes of the contradictory white mindset, "White commentators attributed similarly mixed qualities to the racial others they purported to help, representing them as dangerously dependent at one moment and all too autonomous the next" (5). As a consequence of such a confused awareness, Bucklin concluded that she must impose stratification, and that a white manager "must be represented in some shape, even if they came in the person of an humble hospital nurse" (69). At this juncture of taking on "overseer" duties, Bucklin refused to question her own white positioning. Later in the narrative, however, she entered into circumstances obliging her to adopt a modicum of awareness that her position of whiteness was inimical to her coworkers and herself.

A slightly different scenario obtained at Point Lookout Hospital, where Bucklin paid lip service to equality but exposed a disturbing inconsistency by maintaining that good conditions for black persons should be contingent on good conditions for white soldiers. As she saw it, a white matron at Point Lookout had encouraged women nurses to treat "the contrabands" better than the soldiers, and Bucklin took umbrage at such circumstances. She argued for a kind of pernicious relativity, implying that black persons didn't deserve good food because they weren't used to it: the soldiers "suffer from want of ordinary diet, and saw better food distributed to negroes, with whom corn-bread and bacon had been luxurious living" (115).[15]

In a subsequent incident, Bucklin experienced a change in her outlook when she took time to see the sights in Alexandria, Virginia, recording her first visceral revulsion to slavery. Her trip occurred relatively soon after the Emancipation Proclamation, and as she surveyed a building that had held enslaved people, she wrote that "a slave pen still stood within the city's limits, with auction block standing about it" (131). Registering the suffering experienced at that location, Bucklin felt deep regret for the bondspeople's physical and emotional misery, especially in hearing the stories of the forced separation of families. The same building that had held enslaved people now housed freedpeople, "huddled together" in "poverty" (130), surely an abominable depiction of life on either side of the Emancipation Proclamation, where legal liberty looked only slightly different than slavery.

Bucklin reported an additional, complicating perception, though, when she noted that the ex-bondspeople evidenced "a strange sense of freedom," being guarded as they were by marching Union soldiers: "They felt, where feeling was possible, where it had not been crushed out by life-long bondage, that *they* stood between the combatants, the prize for which they were contending" (130–31). Bucklin offered a contorted and many-faceted perception of their perception, first of all questioning whether they could feel at all—an unfortunate phrase that may have been demeaning but also may have been meant to emphasize that the condition of slavery suppressed feeling altogether, as some nineteenth-century slave narratives report. Further, though, she also contemplated for a moment a new, black point of view: she intuited a "strange sense of freedom" on the part of former slaves who understood the devastating economic value assigned them by white Southerners (and albeit in a different context, by white Northerners, who fixed economic assumptions in the word "contraband"). That the bondspeople saw themselves as a "prize" fought over by Northern and Southern forces showed a trenchant wisdom in their firsthand knowledge that the war was indeed fought over enslaved people, as recent histories such as those by David Blight and Adam Goodheart have reasserted.

Bucklin's view that freedpeople held a singular "sense of freedom" became vexed, however, when she considered that the Alexandria "slave pen" was used simultaneously as a holding tank for white Union soldiers who were military offenders. The army had converted the enclosure to incarcerate soldiers who had been detained, as Bucklin saw it, for "trifling offences, [and] were put under guard in that loathsome pen, when the very dust was alive with vermin" (131). Like the instance at Point Lookout, in which Bucklin argued for preferential treatment for white soldiers regarding food, she argued in this case for better accommodations for white soldiers than for freedpeople and was offended that a former slave "pen" was used to jail white military men.

A later incident cued Bucklin to reorient her outlook and to grant that her experience was shaped by white privilege, even though she previously had been mostly unaware of it. In this circumstance she was forced to admit that the Union soldiers she championed so vigorously now included black men as well, and that her beloved privates—the end-all justification for her own position as nurse—suddenly defied a white-only categorization. After leaving White House on the Pamunkey on a march, she reported that "the first colored wounded I had ever seen filled these old buildings" (282), and described their wounds of "gashed lips," and faces and bodies "covered with gore." Bucklin followed these graphic descriptions with a brief sentence: "These poor fellows were evidently suffering acutely" (283). The sentence showed her sympathy but also carried a disjunctive note with the word "evidently," an adverb she never would have pinned to suffering white soldiers. The slippage exposed Bucklin's difficulty in accepting full status for freedmen and her lingering reticence in conceding equality; still, she took a step toward challenging her intolerant views, given that she granted that their sacrifice equaled that of all soldiers. If she recognized sacrifice and valorized patriotism, she had to credit her honorable rank-and-file soldier as being black as well as a white.

Bucklin continued to amplify this awareness in the last segments of the book, particularly as she served black soldiers at Point of Rocks Hospital in Virginia. This institution, more camp than hospital, had rough accommodations, as Bucklin described them, including canvas roofs, dirt floors, and sleeping spaces so cold the patients' toes sometimes froze. In these buildings, "all soldiers, black and white, were brought to be divested of their torn, bloody uniforms, and to have their swarms of greybacks and their wounds attended to" (333).[16] Working in the "log stockades [that] were principally filled with colored men, wounded on picket, or in the charge on the enemy's works" (333), she came to regard black soldiers' suffering as hardly "apparent," like she had stated before, but as altogether undeniable. Bucklin took pains to declare at more than one point that "white and black were treated alike—both occupying the tents and wooden wards" (337), though by this she did not mean that the troops were integrated, as she clarified that there existed a "white men's ward" (341) and a "colored ward" (342). Overall, the facility had primitive buildings but had a policy of food in abundance, so that the nurses served good meals to their patients "irrespective of color or of State" (334).

In the main, Bucklin embraced patriotic and to some extent antislavery rhetoric to describe these patients as men who did the difficult work of American citizens and soldiers, dedicated to performing the duties of upholding liberty for family and nation. Like Woolsey and Powers, she admired the devout character of the freedmen, noting their reserve as they said devotions under their blankets in bed, their profound investment in the war, and their dedication to family. Bucklin respected abolitionist literacy programs, spending time at Point of Rocks caring for black troops and teaching them to read: "I was exceedingly interested in these men—many of whom had just been liberated from bondage, and were fighting to retain for themselves and children the newly acquired boon of liberty" (337).

Bucklin may have attempted to evoke in her description of Point of Rocks an idyll of democracy where all were welcome and civil. The following statement about black soldiers included an opening that sounded almost utopic, but the ending recalled inequality: "They were universally polite and defferential [*sic*] to me, again and again expressing their gratitude for the good care which northern women gave them, by the remark, 'Jest as if we had white faces missus'" (337–38). The glaring race differential compressed in this remark posed "white" as categorically good and deserving; however, it may be that from the black soldier's perspective—given that white soldiers indeed were usually treated better—that it made sense to thank a white nurse for treating him "as if" he were white, because it acknowledged relatively fair treatment. The black soldier's color reference may also have been a kind of Signifying used to maximize his medical care as he negotiated his way through a new and unfamiliar hospital system that included white women nurses.

At Point of Rocks, Bucklin tended to a wounded and dying black soldier whose "good death" preponderated in serenity over other deathbed scenes in her narrative. The freedman soldier confided to Bucklin his astute reading of the doctor's tone of voice, which foretold probable death, a conclusion Bucklin had not perceived. The soldier was right, however. His suffering was immense, his pain "so intense" that "the five blankets on his bed were wet to the topmost one" (339), and very near the day of his death he requested music, saying to Bucklin, "'How I would like to have the ladies come and sing in the ward to-night'" (339). She arranged it, and after hearing the music he "exhorted all to follow Christ," turning to say to those at his bedside, "'Don't you see the angels all around my bed, waiting for my soul?'" (340).

In this good death, Bucklin drew on the narrative strategy of showing the nurse facilitating a good death, but in this case the death was presented at least partly to show racial equality. The soldier was not surrounded by a circle of family but was attended by a circle of proxies, comprising other patients and nurses who formed a diverse group of black and white people. The deathbed scene drew on the Victorian, Christian expectations of the time, including an iconography of angels. The man gave a lock of hair to be dispensed to a survivor, and also gave Bucklin a silver ring to send home to his mother, along with the lock of hair. When he asked about his burial, Bucklin told him, "'You shall be buried as well as any of them'" (340), out of kindness neglecting to say that "any of them"—white or black—were simply rolled in their blankets and interred.

In further episodes at Point of Rocks, Bucklin maneuvered through bureaucratic channels to help another black soldier in her ward who wondered if "'a colored man could get a furlough'" (341). Neither he nor she knew if such a request had been granted before, but she pursued the matter to secure it for him, and he was granted permission to visit his wife; later, when their daughter was born, they named her Sophronia. Bucklin continued to show that her compassion had deepened when she took up a collection of money for another freedman soldier whose family, through several cruel turns of wartime events, had been reduced to begging because "he had not been paid in eleven months" (343). Knowing firsthand that the withholding of his pay was categorically not because he was "naturally indolent," as in her initial assessment of the women at the laundry, Bucklin championed his cause.

No circumstance showed the alteration in Bucklin's outlook so well as her occupation at a second laundry operation, at Point of Rocks, where once again Bucklin was put in charge: "Each night I sprinkled and folded the clothes for six or eight contraband girls to iron the next day, giving to each one hundred linen sheets" (350). By contrast with the experience at Thirteenth Street Hospital a couple years prior, her opinion of freedwomen had altered: "The girls, who worked in the linen-room under my superintendence, were very quick at their tasks, and all were more intelligent than I had supposed it possible for them to be, having just emerged from a life bondage" (350). She was able to observe the workers' strengths and blamed any weaknesses or lack of education on their former enslavement.

One woman in particular, named Celia, engaged Bucklin's attention: "All but one was very obedient, and she was one of the neatest and smartest of them, but fancied, as freedom had been given them, they were entitled to their support without work" (350–51). She seemed almost to admire Celia all the more for her disobedience—a characteristic easy to imagine Bucklin valuing. While she required Celia to attend work to earn her six dollars per month, she also attempted to win her over in personal ways, such as calling the young woman into her room after overhearing that she planned to wed her sweetheart, a black corporal, and suggesting that Bucklin herself "'make a wedding'" for them (351). Delighted, the bride-to-be consulted with her fiancé and agreed to the arrangement, after which Bucklin decorated the linen-room with chandeliers and wildflowers, procuring "two kinds of cake, some apples, and a pail full of lemonade, inviting as guests the surgeons and their wives, the ward masters, cooks, women nurses, and Chaplain Hager, who was to officiate" (351). Soon after Bucklin organized this party of mixed races and classes, Celia stopped in to say good-bye, as her soldier husband had received orders to remove to Texas (with his wife).[17] Celia's action of stopping to say farewell intimated a mutual regard between the women.

Soon after the war, Bucklin found it necessary to defend her newfound interracial associations in a remarkable meeting in which she felt her loyalties divided between white, upper-class women and black working women. She gathered with a half-dozen white women "near where the contrabands were ironing" (367), and the black women spoke at a volume such that the white women expressed disapproval: "Each race saw the other, and the working girls, feeling indignant and having a keen appreciation of their newly acquired independence, talked so loudly amongst themselves that we heard every word" (367). The freedwomen spoke loudly so as to signal their emancipation to the white women, and the white women urged Bucklin to stop the black women's independent behavior. They pressured her to silence the talk, especially when the freedwomen started to criticize the white women and praise Bucklin: "One said, 'There isn't a decent woman in there, only Miss Bucklin,' to which the others assented in strong terms" (367). The white women threatened to leave if Bucklin refused to subdue the workers, and finally departed, "highly offended because I did not 'slap the wenches on their mouths'" (368).

The white women's presumption of position through whiteness suggested a close alliance with the violent position of the slaveholder, a presumption emphatically reflected in their expectation that Bucklin physically punish the black workers. The white women imagined their status to be assailed by the black women's insistence on freedom of expression, and Bucklin proved her awareness of the dynamic by defending them: "I felt sure that my ironing girls appeared far superior to the snuff'eating women—and that they best knew to what indignities they had been subjected under their hands" (368). Bucklin acknowledged that the ex-bondswomen "knew best," validating and honoring their knowledge of their personal experience as an essential right. Knowing that they were highly capable of forming their own perceptions, she found them more commendable by far than the white women, about whom she delivered this acrimonious aside: "I will add that it was a warm May day, and these [white] women were dressed in muslins and furs, with ribbons of various colors on their heads" (368). She offered the fashion statement as a final commentary on the matter, the accouterments of entitlement speaking volumes about the white women's ignorance of real work. Bucklin's final admiration of the black women as exemplars of American decency and moral character demonstrated a significant shift from her early posture of assuming white power and privilege to a later adoption of a more inclusive view, in which she embraced the dignity of her black coworkers.

Bucklin's narrative presented a larger panorama of interracial interactions than did the work of other nurse narrators studied here. She presented, too, more various means of the types of dissent available to her. Framing the cause of freedom from the beginning of her memoir by referring to the Declaration of Independence and the Seneca Falls declaration, she clearly articulated gender equality and developed a discourse that drew from these sources to defend Civil War working women. Within this framework she advanced the female nurse's claim to legitimacy as a person who offered valuable service to the Union. Bucklin's advocacy steeled her to fight first for working-class privates and to dissent when they were mistreated—an advocacy she extended eventually to black as well as white soldiers, and to black women as well as black men, giving careful attention to the freedmen and freedwomen at Point of Rocks Hospital. As she said of the black women with whom she worked, they owned "a keen appreciation of their newly acquired independence" (367).

As a relief worker alongside rank-and-file soldiers, Bucklin was inspired to undertake labor in the name of nation. She militated for others, garnering the assurance to herald rights for those with less access to power than the officials. She wielded a patriotic discourse to show devotion to the rank-and-file, which included the diverse soldiers and workers whose earnest, forthright actions she honored. In the end, Bucklin judged people on their ability to contribute clean, hard industry to their country, regardless of gender and class and, at least in the latter parts of her narrative, regardless of race. She aligned herself with the workers. Those who did not do their part, she took to task.

Echo answers, 'when!' (69)

CHAPTER SEVEN

Julia S. Wheelock's *The Boys in White*

Narrative Construction

Julia Wheelock entered the work of nursing when she journeyed from Ionia, Michigan, to Alexandria, Virginia, after hearing that her brother, Orville Wheelock, had been wounded and his leg amputated in the Battle of Chantilly in September 1862. She worked as a teacher in Ionia, and as she was listening to the recitation of one of her students three days before the end of the school year, she received news about her brother's injury from a little girl on the school doorstep. The next day, Wheelock, her sister-in-law Anna, and Anna's sister left for Virginia to attempt to find Orville, intending to nurse him back to health, only to discover upon arrival that he had passed away. Julia Wheelock stayed on to nurse others.[1]

In Washington, DC, waiting for a nursing position to open, Wheelock saw injured soldiers from the onslaught at Antietam crowd the makeshift hospital inside the DC Patent Office, witnessing "for the first time the wounded as they came from the battlefield" (31). She and another woman distributed cakes and crackers to these patients, an experience that overwhelmed her: "The sight was too much for me; I was completely unnerved . . . I returned to my room to weep over the sufferings I was powerless to alleviate" (32). Her previously unremarkable life was transformed and, as Julia Pferdehirt observes about Wheelock and other nurses from sheltered middle- and upper-class families, she would be sheltered "no more" (43). In Wheelock's own words from a slightly different context, she experienced a veritable "exchange of worlds."

She found a position as agent for the Michigan Relief Association, engaging in work similar to that of Georgeanna Woolsey, the latter serving a national commission, and Wheelock a state association. Despite the fact that both were relief workers, though, the parameters of the two women's narratives differed markedly, Woolsey writing her narrative after nursing intensively for a short period of time in the aftermath of one of the largest conflagrations of the war, and Wheelock writing hers over a period of three years, from different sites in the Washington area. Julia Wheelock eventually worked in twenty-five hospitals and attended to soldiers from three major battles surrounding the area—Antietam, September 1862; Fredericksburg, December 1862; and Gettysburg, July 1863, among others. Both did relief work, but Woolsey's relationship with her audience in 1863 was predicated on the need to urge readers to make donations, whereas Wheelock's, in 1870, was to voice grief over the war casualties.

Despite addressing national issues, Wheelock's narrative garnered mostly regional reviews and local attention. In the *Detroit Free Press*, for instance, the author of an article entitled "From the Fifth Infantry" praised Wheelock among three Michigan women nurses, asking readers to "allow me to make some mention of heroines in the field, Mrs. Brainard, the mother of every Michigan soldier, Miss Julia Wheelock, the kind benefactress and untiring friend of our men, and last, but not least, Miss Annie Etheridge, who is, and for the last three years has always been in the front" (August 10, 1864; 3). The *Jackson Citizen Patriot*, another Michigan paper, praised Wheelock's book in terms of Alcott's, as "a collection of hospital sketches," and appreciated the no-nonsense tone: Wheelock "ventures no flights of imagination, but gives a truer insight of hospital

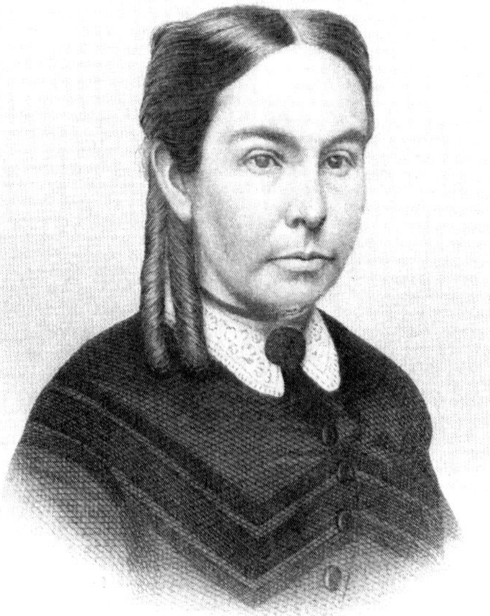

Julia Wheelock
Julia Wheelock,
The Boys in White, 1870

life than has hitherto been presented in any work we have seen" (June 24, 1879; 5). The *Jackson Citizen Patriot* exhibited state pride in its reporting, favoring the local girl who gave service to her state over others.[2] Wheelock's audience probably comprised primarily Michigan readers. Her narrative was aimed at least in part toward their concerns, as another report from the *Jackson Citizen Patriot* showed in exhorting readers to buy Wheelock's book, which "deserves well of public patronage and should have an extensive sale, especially among relatives and friends of Michigan soldiers, in whose behalf her labors were mainly given" (June 24, 1870; 5). The article made clear that Wheelock would soon "canvass the city" for the express purpose of sales.

In Washington, DC, Wheelock and another Michigan woman were "the only regularly employed visiting agents" (36) from the state, and under the aegis of the relief agency Wheelock did "what she could to comfort other Michigan boys who would otherwise not have received much kindly attention from an overworked medical staff" (Gillespie,

Andersonvilles of the North 219). In order to meet with soldiers the two women undertook the immense task of tracking down each of the men in a hospital system characterized by "changes which were constantly taking place by death, discharges, transfers, furloughs, new arrivals, and returns to duty, which were of almost daily occurrence" (38). Serving Michigan soldiers in fourteen hospitals occupying twenty different buildings where, in each hospital, "two to fifteen hundred patients" stayed (37), the two women were kept extraordinarily busy. Over the course of the narrative Wheelock visited patients, for example, in Washington; Alexandria, Virginia; Baltimore; Harrisburg, Pennsylvania; and elsewhere, sometimes traveling to the front, as to Falmouth, Massachusetts, "with nearly four thousand pounds of hospital stores" (83).

National and state relief workers were of enormous importance to the war effort, given that at the onset of the conflict the United States had no preexisting readiness for war, and its extent and duration had not been anticipated. In her introduction to *Hospital Sketches*, Bessie Jones writes, "before Sumter there was not a single general army hospital in the country"; furthermore, "the Medical Department had no unified staff, no nurses, no diet charts, no provisions for clothing" (Introduction xxliii). Wheelock carried needed items to soldiers in various hospitals: "cooked tomatoes or stewed fruit . . . chicken broth, pickles, butter, cheese, jelly, tea hot from the stove . . . oranges, lemons, and fresh fruit," as well as such nonfood items as "shirts, drawers, socks, slippers, dressing-gowns, towels and handkerchiefs, also stationery and reading-matter" (38). Exposing the government's inability at times to supply even the most basic articles for wounded soldiers, relief agencies pitched in with provisions.

Working for a state agency in some ways rendered Wheelock's job more onerous than working at a single hospital because it put her in transit among various locales, but it also may have given her some personal agency as a more or less lone operative. Writing that Michigan soldiers were "largely represented" (124) among the hospitals, Wheelock often thought of her "home" as the 26th Michigan Volunteers, and took pleasure in keeping track of regiment members' adventures and difficulties; inevitably, she also tracked their losses. She made the rounds of other Michigan regiments as well, and assisted many soldiers not from her

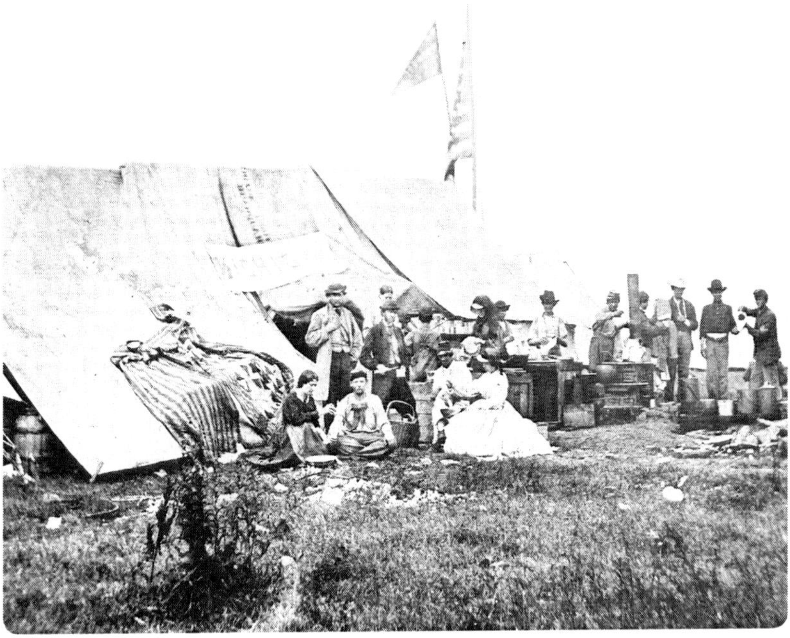

Michigan and Pennsylvania Relief Associations, White House Landing, Virginia

Courtesy of the Library of Congress

home state, too—"any and all, who appealed for aid" (166).[3] More than once she took pains to clarify, "I could not turn a deaf ear to a soldier's wants" (166); for instance, on one visit she served chicken soup and crackers, affirming that in doling out the food, "I made no distinction, but gave to all as far as my supplies would go" (192).

This chapter examines three facets of Julia Wheelock's narrative: dissent, narrative construction, and the interrogation of suffering as focused on grief and memory. Through these facets *The Boys in White* addresses some of the major considerations of discourse in *Civil War Nurse Narratives.* First, regarding dissent, Wheelock's position with the state relief agency in Washington, far from the center of operations in Michigan, enabled her to avoid being under the direct supervision of a controlling federal or hospital administrator and thus may have given her increased opportunity to be assertive in conflicts with hospital officials; accordingly, Wheelock's narrative, "one of the more informative accounts" (Massey 187), showed dissent with authorities at several impasses. Next, regarding composition, access to Wheelock's materials allows us to track the choices she made as she constructed her prose, revised expressly toward drawing in the reader. We can see how she consulted her diary, in which she recorded the daily activities of her service, in order to construct the narrative of *The Boys in White*. To examine her papers, including diary, manuscript, and scrapbook, is to discover how Wheelock made the shift from private to public expression. Finally, regarding grief and memory, Wheelock invested the title trope, "the boys in white" with the means to represent both personal and public loss. Wheelock registered bereavement in conscious and unconscious ways, mirroring an American society in the process of coping with war exhaustion, postwar trauma, and the rebuilding of a society in the aftermath of fractured families, ideologies, and institutions.

IF WORKING FOR a state relief agency gave Julia Wheelock more latitude for dissent, she nonetheless seemed inclined to act assertively even before being employed. She seldom hesitated to intercede when she saw the need, as in an instance near the beginning of the memoir, when she and her companions journeyed east in the hopes of finding Orville Wheelock. The three women needed passes to Alexandria but found themselves blocked by a sign announcing, "'No passes granted on Sunday'" (16), and waited in an office where supplicants for passes were all summarily refused exemption from the Sunday rule. When it came turn for Wheelock's party, the women met the marshal "tremblingly" and faced him "with more deference than is meet should be paid to mortals," but still received an unyielding response: "'Why do you ask us to violate orders?'" (16–17). As spokesperson for the three women, Wheelock portrayed herself as using a discourse of indirection, engaging his blocking question with a question that opened the situation out: "'Will no circumstances justify you in granting a pass to-day?'" (17). With this interchange, the marshal allowed them to explain the extenuating circumstances involving their injured family member, watched them "closely to see whether we were deceiving him," and finally permitted them the passes needed. It is worth noting that in her diary, often very detailed, Wheelock recorded only a brief statement about the episode: "We then went to the Provost Marshals to get a pass to go across the Potomac. It was against their rules to give passes on sunday [*sic*]—but under the circumstances they granted us one" (Wheelock Collection 1:2, Sept 14, 1862). The diary account featured no dialogue and no initiative taken by Wheelock and proved notably less dramatic than the scene presented in the book. It appears that it was important to Wheelock to demonstrate to her readers that as a woman she could muster the communication necessary to negotiate difficult circumstances.

In a second instance of speaking out, Wheelock's firm manner served her well in dealing with the authorities of Camp Convalescent. Relatively early in the narrative, one of her passions became the care of the men at Camp Convalescent, a large area outside Alexandria set aside for patients who ostensibly had recuperated sufficiently to leave the hospital. Wheelock found, however, that many of the patients had not recovered, and that the camp lacked the basic necessities. Conditions of utter "wretchedness" prevailed: "Here were from ten to fifteen thousand soldiers—not simply the convalescent, but the sick and dying—many of them destitute, with not even a blanket or an overcoat, having little or no wood" (39). As did many commenters at the time, Wheelock called the place "Camp Misery," comparing it even to Southern prison camps, not in general conditions but in execrable particulars, the more reprehensible because Camp Convalescent was under Northern control: "Think of men sick with fever, pneumonia, or chronic diarrhea, eating raw pork and lying upon the cold, damp ground, with only one blanket, and, it may be, none, and the wonder will be, not that they died, but that any recovered" (39).

Others gave similar accounts. The Christian Commission Report of 1863 expressed abhorrence at the conditions: "The suffering was unparalleled and appalling. Despondency and despair, aided by cold, hunger, filth, vermin, and disease, settled heavily upon thousands of hearts" (United States Christian Commission 50). The camp housed 22,000 men and consisted of three disparate groups: the parole camp, "a great gathering-place of our own men taken and paroled by the rebels"; the straggler camp for men waiting to be reassigned; and the camp proper, "where the men from various hospitals were sent as soon as they so far recovered as to admit of it" (49). In 1895, Noah Brooks described the "infamous" location as a holding place for honorable soldier convalescents along with those of questionable character, the "'bummers,' deserters, and stragglers—the riffraff of the Federal and Confederate armies" (Brooks, *Washington in Lincoln's Time* 6).

Wheelock arrived at the camp on one occasion with forty-two homemade pies, the pastries proving, not surprisingly, to be a hit, but to the point of almost causing a little riot: "The moment it was known there were pies in camp our ambulance would be surrounded, and we, the occupants, literally taken prisoners; some begging for themselves, others for a sick comrade who was unable to leave the quarters. At such times how earnestly I wished that the miracle of the "loaves and fishes" might be repeated" (44–45). Wheelock often baked through the evenings so that she could supply patients with fresh food the next day, including the Camp Convalescent men among her rounds. The men also benefited from her deliveries of quilts, underclothing, towels, handkerchiefs, socks, flannel shirts, and other items. She reported that though handing out needed items at the beginning of the visit was a pleasure, there was always a cause for sorrow at the end, for whatever she took, there was never enough, and the men would jostle each other as she ran out of goods.

Such disheartening experiences probably caused her to act even more directly. Soon after the pie distribution episode, she made a dramatic (and ironic) announcement that she had kidnapped some men, that she "fell in with a practice which I had always greatly abhorred, that of kidnapping—not black men however, but white men—soldiers" (55). Momentarily situating her action in terms of the execrable practice of slavery, she secured her readers' attention, then brought them back to the actions of relief work, the "kidnapping," of course, having not only the full consent but the benediction of those who were "stolen." Discovering several Michigan men too sick to recover at the camp, she attempted to procure authorization for their return to a hospital where they properly belonged. On this mission Wheelock was met with formidable red tape in a series of parries with officials: she was referred to Colonel Belknap, the commanding officer, who referred her to Dr. Jacobs, the surgeon-in-charge, who sent her to Dr. Robertson, surgeon of the admitting hospital, who handed her over to Dr. Summers, the physician in charge of Dr. Robertson's hospital, who passed her off to the medical director in Washington.

Knowing she wouldn't find the medical director at the capital because it was the weekend, she found herself in a position somewhat similar to the one at the outset of the journey when passes seemed to be unavailable because of the Sunday prohibition. Wheelock had then created the terms for the results she desired and would this time, too, but added one more potentially precarious tack: when she made her case she decided to omit the need for permission at the starting point of her mission. That is to say, she consulted with Dr. Robertson, who agreed that he would ensure patients' admittance to his hospital if Wheelock could get them out of Camp Convalescent. Assured of clear passage on the receiving end, she assumed responsibility for the starting point, procuring an ambulance on the weekend and rounding up six soldiers whom she transported out of the camp with no permission from the camp official. She then delivered them to the hospital, after which one very sick man soon died, his fatality a sad testimony to how grievously ill the men were. The others recovered, however, and at least one of them credited her afterward with saving his life.

She kidnapped again. On another occasion Wheelock brought three sick men after dark to McVey Hospital, only to realize that the surgeon-in-charge was no longer the same man, and the hospital would not permit access. Her only option was to confront the new surgeon, Dr. Curtis, face-to-face, and accordingly, she ran "up-stairs to his office and related what I had done" (70). Surprisingly, the surgeon allowed the infraction, instructing her not to do it again, but kindly offering to receive as many sick men as she wished to admit in the future, so long as he knew about it beforehand.[4]

On the whole, kind doctors were in the majority in Wheelock's experience, but many of their well-intentioned actions met with bureaucratic obstructions, so she learned to challenge "the intricate windings of 'red tape'" (69).[5] In the case of Camp Convalescent, however, she suspected actions more inimical than those simply due to red tape, actions of gross mismanagement or even extortion of resources: "There was blame attached to some one—a fearful neglect of duty somewhere" (78).[6] Congress finally recognized the manifold abuses by the administrators of the camp in the Senate resolution of December 4, 1862, which stated the following: "Whereas it is reported that many abuses exist in connexion [*sic*] with the administration of 'Camp Convalescent,' near Alexandria, and until they are corrected the health and lives of the thousands of our brave soldiers there stationed will continue to be endangered" (Reports 549). The Congressional deliberations resulted in an order on December 9, 1862, that barracks would be constructed at the camp to alleviate some of the dangerous conditions (553). Wheelock noted in her narrative that in January 1863, such construction had begun.

Personally aware of the windings of red tape and the outrages of neglect, Wheelock took on authorities and exhibited a composure that helped remove obstacles to her patients' recoveries. Like Bucklin, Wheelock used specific forms of dissent that included interpretation, appeal, and noncompliance in the kidnapping episodes. She did not use direct confrontation at first, but saved that for later, in clashes with officials at an Alexandria hospital and St. Paul's Hospital. At an Alexandria hospital she met a particularly contentious physician who denied her admittance, demanding that she first receive written permission from Dr. Edwin Bently, the surgeon in charge. The fact of being denied entrance "was something new," and Wheelock, who had heard reports of suspicious treatment of "our boys" at that particular hospital, began "to think there was some truth to the reports" (129). She argued with the physician that Dr. Bently's office was a mile away, and he countered that he himself would go, but she must wait until he returned. In direct contradiction, Wheelock said, "'But I can't wait, doctor; I shall go through the wards while you are gone'" (130). To this, surprisingly, he acceded, and she made the rounds, surveying some further conditions that convinced her there were grounds for the negative reports. At a later time, she took the conflict with the doctor one step further by calling on Dr. Bently herself, and he corroborated that she did not need a pass to enter the hospital and furthermore, that she had full access to it: "'And you tell the doctor for me, that you have the privilege of visiting my hospitals as often as you wish, and at such times as best suit your convenience'" (130).

In the same Alexandria hospital, Wheelock one night brought "two large bottles of blackberry-wine" slated for two particular patients, but a guard at the door stopped her and prevented entry, saying he had orders to admit no one, "not even the President of the United States" (131). Wheelock's solution was to go to the sergeant of the guard, who allotted her the permission she needed, after which she left the wine to be administered if the doctor deemed it helpful, then exited before "his 'highness' returned" (131). Afterward she learned that the surgeon in charge had become enraged about the blackberry wine and thrown one bottle out the window, though the other bottle was saved by a patient who hid it under his pillow, to administer later.

On yet another, more serious occasion involving the same doctor, two patients in dire condition needed discharges to go home, and when Wheelock inquired about them the surgeon informed her that he had filed the appropriate papers. Some weeks later, however, she found that the men were still there and she confronted him, asking, "'if he could account for the delay'" (132). The surgeon responded a second time that he had sent the needed papers, but after the passage of yet more time the men had not been discharged. At this point Wheelock decided to visit the medical director in Washington, where she was informed after two close examinations of the books that the papers had never arrived, after which she went directly to the Secretary of War's office to expose the abuse. Soon afterward, the culpable surgeon was removed from his post, and very soon after that, the two patients received permission to return to their homes. One died soon after.

One final act of dissent occurred in an encounter at St. Paul's Hospital, where Wheelock ran afoul of a surgeon who accosted her rudely, demanding to know what she had in a bowl she held, to which she replied that it contained tea she had brought for "that New York man over there; he can't drink the tea made here, so I bring him some occasionally—any objections, doctor?" He answered that he didn't object to the tea, but objected to her, and turned on his heel. The New York soldier then "burst into tears and begged me to 'come again, while others expressed their regrets, saying, 'The doctor is real mean to act so'" (60–1). The soldiers professed the benefit of receiving Wheelock's care, a camaraderie the nurse narrators portrayed as a confirmation of their good work. Wheelock assured the men that she would settle her differences with the doctor so she could return, then revisited St. Paul's to request that the doctor give her "an explanation of his strange conduct toward me" (63). He answered that she was a nurse assigned to work at Wolfe Street Hospital, and had "no business to interfere with mine; and I don't want you to come here any more" (64). Wheelock informed him point blank that he was "mistaken," because she did not "belong" to any one hospital or another, proudly avowing her relative autonomy, at which defense, he capitulated immediately, apologized, and welcomed her to visit "his" hospital anytime.[7] Wheelock forgave the doctor, though she couldn't help but add a maxim for her reader: "How much better it would be to treat every one with true politeness which costs nothing, and thereby save ourselves much deep mortification" (64). In this incisive interchange, she exculpated women workers, argued for their right to offer feedback on the work of nursing, and defended their prerogative to act as exemplars of rectitude.

Wheelock portrayed herself as being made of stern stuff, initiating encounters with superiors based on her commitment to the mission of the Union soldiers' well-being, asserting that intercession for patients "was but a small part of our work (145). She used a politics of intercession to temper what might otherwise have been seen as aggressive, impudent actions and, on the whole, balanced dissent and tact. For instance, in relating an early contretemps with a surgeon over what a patient should eat, she showed her readers that she eventually "complied with the surgeon's wishes" (53), but couldn't help adding, "I always made it a rule to do so, believing that their judgment was superior to mine, or at least ought to be, though I sometimes saw those whom I thought knew less" (53). Wheelock used a rhetoric of indirection, mixing in a bit of deliberate irony. Her brand of disputation usually fell short of blatant opposition, even as she trusted her own power of discernment. Upon such nuances she built a kind of platform of intervention from which she could justify the most audacious dissent. For instance, she conducted the "kidnappings" soon after she had "complied with the surgeon's wishes." In these ways she nodded to her female audience.

ACCESS TO WHEELOCK'S PAPERS allows us to examine her process of narrative construction and deduce the means by which she appealed to a readership. Wheelock affirmed that her narrative had been transposed from journal entries and "condensed," before it was published and "thrown into the lap of the public and of my friends'" (v).[8] An inveterate diarist during and after the war, she kept a daily journal, with only herself as recipient: "the journal was kept for my personal benefit, and not for publication" (v). Wheelock recorded daily entries from September 10, 1862 through December 31, 1867, in two oblong books with multicolored, marbled covers.[9] Registering day-to-day impressions, she wrote variously in pencil and ink, each entry of a different length, some longer than a page and some terse, as for example this one-sentence entry: "Sewed nearly all day" (1:5, Oct 26, 1862). Many parts of the book, *The Boys in White*, borrowed whole phrases and sentences from the diary, while other parts elaborated on diary passages and experimented with modes of expression. Though she often followed her diary relatively closely, Wheelock at other times added altogether new sections, in all cases reshaping material into a rhetoric suitable for audience reception.

The episode in which Wheelock prepared to leave Michigan and travel to Virginia exemplifies the contrast between diary and book, the differences highlighting the narrative decisions she made. For instance, in the brief description of receiving notice at the schoolhouse about her brother's wound, Wheelock wrote in her diary: "At ½ past 3'o'clock Taisie Stone called and ~~wish~~ wished to see me . . ." (1;1 Sept 10, 1862).[10] She recorded this with no further embroidery, but in the book chose to frame the scene, telling the reader that the news came from a young person: "A child is made the bearer of the sad message" (10). Such a choice accentuated the sentimental quality of the scene, given that a small girl delivered the momentous news, and Wheelock amplified the effect with phrases like "a little girl steps upon the threshold," and "there is a gentle tap at the door" (10). Both of these additions underscored the fact that news of the crisis came from the mouth of an innocent child, thus rendering the moment of receiving the news more poignant for the audience.

Wheelock displayed a relatively clipped version of her reaction to the news in the diary, in which she took no heroic measures but, pragmatically, began to sew: "I hastily closed my school, and with hurried and anxious steps went to Mr. Ritts, to assist in making some clothes for Sister Anna, who was going to start for Washington the next day— " (1:1, Sept 10, 1862). In the more sentimental book, however, she decided immediately to accompany her sister-in-law to Washington because her "womanly heart" told her she needed to ensure her brother would "not suffer alone" (10). Whereas the diary account depicted Wheelock following the dictates of efficiency in readying travel clothes for her sister-in-law, the book account showed Wheelock's "womanly heart" hurrying to her sister-in-law and her brother. Wheelock invented scenes in the book that were moved by emotion, the more directly to reach a female audience steeped in similarly toned reading materials.

She embellished many such scenes in this way, as for instance, when the three women—Wheelock, Anna, and Anna's sister—undertook the journey to Washington and along the way encountered new landscapes. Whereas the diary reported in pedestrian prose their crossing of Lake Erie, the book elaborated on crossing the waters as if Wheelock could see imagined war scenes against the backdrop of Lake Erie: "the battle-field with its thousands of mangled forms, the dead and dying, and all the horrors connected with such scenes of carnage, are spread out before us" (12). Wheelock utilized the nurse narrative staple of depicting the scene of travel, including this devastating foreshadowing, which was perhaps cribbed from Alcott (who also wrote of mangled forms during her travel sequence). Wheelock augmented the travel scene to guide her readers to anticipate moments very like those she would witness in the military hospital when the actual "bloody, mangled forms" of the wounded arrived from Antietam (31). Similarly, Wheelock chronicled details of the scenery between Pittsburgh and Harrisburg, both diary and book describing the view as "sublime," though in the former she admitted that "we went through the famous tunnel in the Alleghany mountains in the night, so lost much of the novelty of the place" (1:1, Sept 10, 1862), and in the latter she expounded on the darkness of the tunnel as a vision of extreme mutability, "where in a moment midnight darkness succeeds to the brightness of noon, producing feelings—one might imagine—akin to a sudden exchange of worlds" (12). This last phrase underlined the sudden shift from civilian to military life and involved the reader—as "one might imagine"—in a conversational relationship.

Arguably the most essential scene in the book—a scene that included the first iteration of the title phrase "boys in white"—was not included in the diary. Only the book offered the scene of an unknown soldier's funeral procession: the three women, on arriving in Alexandria, encouraged to think they would find Orville in the Lyceum, were blocked after only a few steps toward that goal by a funeral. Wheelock's invention of the procession is instrumental for marking her authorial design in writing a public memoir, in which "one of our country's heroes, one of the 'boys in white,' lies in that plain coffin," escorted by fellow soldiers who march, "keeping time with their slow tread to the solemn notes of the 'Dead March'" (20–21). In the middle of their quest for Orville, the women were stopped by the somber ceremony, immediately after which they discovered that the first report of Orville's health was mistaken and that, as an informant reported to them, Orville had actually died soon after the Battle of Chantilly and been buried days before their arrival.

Wheelock's compositional process can be discerned by contrasting examples of diary entries she altered or extended, but it can also be grasped by looking at the manuscript form of the book. Wheelock's manuscript version of *The Boys in White* included revisions later added to the finished volume, revisions that disclose tight stylings in her attentions to audience. For instance, she related in the first sentences of the manuscript that much of her journal "was written late at night, when so wearied by excessive labor, (mental) anxiety, and excitement that I would not unfrequently fall asleep with the pen in my hand" (Manuscript 3). The parentheses around the word "mental" indicate that the word was to be omitted for the final version of the book, which it was. Apparently, Wheelock chose at first to represent mental distress, but on reflection decided to indicate only physical discomfort; she may have perceived her readers as wanting a more mentally certain attitude from a nurse. She also accommodated her readers by making another omission that greatly changed the book. That is, on the next page she enclosed five words in parentheses to slate them for omission, as follows: "Justice, (not only to myself, but) to our noble soldiers demands, that I should here state, that during my hospital and army experience of nearly three years, I was uniformly treated with the utmost courtesy and respect" (Manuscript 4). Originally writing the sentence to declare justice for both herself and the soldiers, the manuscript disavowed overt self-concern by deleting the parenthetical phrase altogether, so that the book sentence read, "Justice to our noble soldiers demands, that I should here state, that during my hospital and army experience of nearly three years, I was uniformly treated with the utmost courtesy and respect" (vi). Hoping to repudiate charges that either female nurses or soldiers behaved in unseemly ways, Wheelock chose to delete "herself" as a way to credit the soldiers alone for protecting her reputation.[11] Self-effacingly she embraced the ideal of the noble common soldier, while remaining discreetly modest, promoting patriotism as she kept female honor intact.

The manuscript version reveals, too, that Wheelock revised the book by adding poetry extracts, thereby contributing a lyrical resonance and rhythmic component to the memoir. She adjoined, for instance, a crucial quatrain to the funeral procession scene described above, with lines that underscored the procession's "slow tread" and "solemn notes of the 'Dead March'" (21). The quatrain echoed the somber moments of the funeral procession scene, as for instance in these lines: "'Aye! Follow his corpse to its last long rest,/With the fife and muffled drum'" (Ms. 26, reverse). Wheelock did not originally include the quatrain in the manuscript but interpolated it later, indicating with an asterisk the inclusion of the poetry, copied on the back of the next manuscript page.[12]

The skill used in making such an addition is commensurate, to a degree, with the artistry of keeping a scrapbook. Wheelock's diary and manuscript demonstrate in direct ways how she deferred to her audience, while her scrapbook, less associated with any final written product, gauged her sense of form in the act of writing. The pastime of keeping a

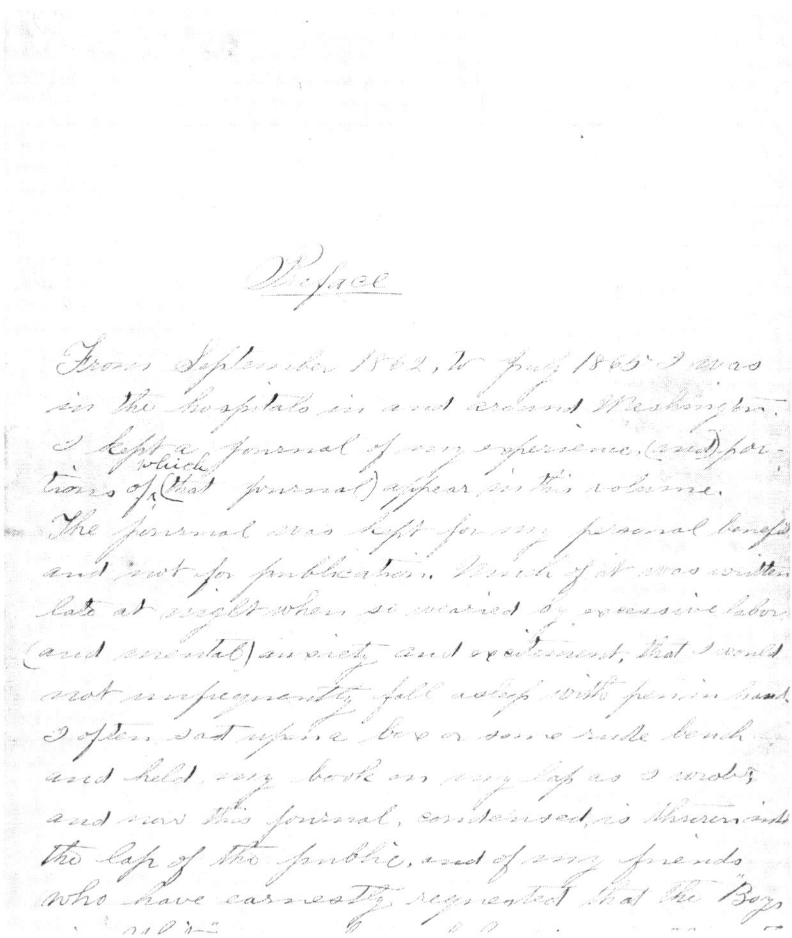
Preface

From September 1862, to July 1865 I was
in the hospitals in and around Washington.
I kept a journal of my experience, (and) por-
tions of (that journal) which appear in this volume.
The journal was kept for my personal benefit
and not for publication. Much of it was written
late at night when so wearied by excessive labor
(and mental) anxiety and excitement, that I would
not unfrequently fall asleep with pen in hand.
I often sat upon a box or some rude bench
and held my book on my lap as I wrote,
and now this journal, condensed, is thrown into
the lap of the public, and of my friends
who have earnestly requested that the Boys

Page from Wheelock Manuscript

Courtesy of the Abraham Lincoln Library and Museum
of Lincoln Memorial University, Harrogate, TN

scrapbook incorporates the ability to arrange magazine and newspaper material—prominently poetry—into an album. In keeping with the standard practice of the time, Wheelock lavished her scrapbook with stanzas of verse, which give us a fresh glimpse into the visualization, preparation, and process behind her work. The scrapbook exhibits the painstaking practice of manually cutting and pasting into a personal album many notable memorial verses of the period.

Wheelock's heavy, oversized scrapbook was a labor of exacting presentation, displaying the typical nineteenth-century symmetry of "sober parallel columns, imitating the newspapers themselves—no cutting loose in wild diagonals, hardly anything sideways, rarely a heading straddling more than a single column" (Garvey, "Imitation").[13] For the most part, the scrapbook conformed to this aesthetic of exacting column arrangement, with a thorough application of magazine and newspaper pages to album pages that left no corners curled or loosened. The work shows the typical scrapbook aesthetic of the period, in "densely covering the pages with clippings" (Garvey, *Writing* 99). (Attesting to her painstaking work, Wheelock's clippings still adhere to the page 150 years later.) Dominated by poems, the scrapbook contains prose, too, usually grouped by subject in several-page batches.

Wheelock's scrapbook may have functioned as a repository for inspiring phrases, a kind of seedbed for ideas from which she could nurture her own points of view.[14] Its ready store of source material argued for a years-long habit of collecting bits of text that aided in the practice of matching epigrammatic expressions with experience.[15] Especially near the end of the album, at the tops or margins of certain poems, handwritten comments such as "Beautiful," "Good," or "Touching" have been added. Also near the end of the scrapbook Wheelock made notations next to several poems, marked in pen with an *x*. For instance, double exes are marked at the top of Alcott's poem, "My Kingdom" (Scrapbook 130).[16]

Several pages in the scrapbook, however, fall outside the realm of usual scrapbooking practice, showing perhaps that Wheelock grew bolder in continuing to arrange her clippings. Particularly in later pages, Wheelock indulged in a somewhat curious variety of placements. For example, in one case, created a few years after the war, she uncharacteristically pasted several types of genres on one page. The page was covered with personal memorabilia, images, a letter, and poems. One of these items, positioned vertically, is a "Reward of Merit" certifying that Susan Wheelock, "The Bearer, receives this as the reward of good behavior and diligent attention to study in school" (Scrapbook 113).[17] Wheelock affixed the Reward of Merit vertically to adjoin a similar reward, also to Susan Wheelock. The letter included on the page, from 1868, was addressed to

"Mr. Hoge, Our Friend and Superintendent," its contents comparing him to "Rock of Ages," and thanking him for his "numerous kindnesses." It was signed by two women, with an added paper bearing seven other names, including Julia Wheelock's. The largest image on the page is a drawing from a publication entitled "The Only Daughter," and the two poems situated beneath it are "Over and Over Again," by Ada Simpson Sherwood, and "The Snow-Storm" by Ralph Waldo Emerson.[18] Having saved visual copies, documents, awards, and poems, she assembled many genres within one page, a collection tantamount to a nineteenth-century version of a multimedia production. Wheelock possessed an active mind, constantly in the habit of compiling thoughts as she combined personal documents, prose, images, and poems. Through her scrapbook she conducted a lively conversation with the media of her day.

AS WE TURN TO a consideration of Wheelock's representation of grief, it is instructive to revisit the fact that the scene of the funeral procession, which Wheelock wrote purposely for *The Boys in White*, was arguably the central scene of the narrative. The three women had taken a few steps toward the Lyceum they thought would lead them to Orville, and were interrupted by the funeral procession of an unknown soldier. Again, the scene locates the point at which Wheelock chose to deliver this specific material to her reader, focusing on the procession of an unidentified soldier, who clearly had not been graced by a good death:

> How unlike a funeral at home! No train of weeping friends follow his bier; yet one of our country's heroes, one of the "boys in white," lies in that plain coffin. He is escorted to his resting-place by perhaps a dozen comrades, who go with unfixed bayonets, and arms reversed, keeping time with their slow tread to the solemn notes of the "Dead March," plaintively executed by some of their number. (20–21)

Immediately after the procession passed, the women were informed that Orville had died days earlier. Stunned, they visited Orville Wheelock's grave, a "turfless mound"—one of almost 300 graves, each marked by a stone, upon which Anna threw herself and sobbed, while Julia Wheelock reminded herself that her brother would rise to heaven. Through this scene Wheelock conditioned her audience to her overarching concern with the nature of grief and memory.

Wheelock had stated that her work was composed in response to friends "who have earnestly requested that 'The Boys in White' be embalmed, as well as the 'Boys in Blue'" (v). She used the word "embalmed" metaphorically when she stated that her friends wished her to preserve, or "embalm," her hospital experiences by writing a book, but she also used the word to honor the war dead by referencing funeral rites, such as that of being "embalmed."[19] By naming her memoir *The Boys in White* she focused on the wounded in the hospitals; both hospitals and trains of wounded flew white flags to indicate they were exempt from attack. The phrase "boys in white" may also have signified departed patients, sometimes wrapped in white blankets after passing away. Like Holstein, Wheelock was preoccupied with the demarcation between life and death and did not hesitate to bring suffering and demise to the forefront; unlike Holstein, she inclined toward offsetting gruesome war deaths with the rhetoric of Christianity and patriotism. The gesture, however, did not always seem to console her, and she seemed often to be of two minds about bereavement. Wheelock addressed mourning from this very early scene, in which she first heard the misinformation that her brother had survived—after which a funeral procession passed—and she then heard that he had not survived. The procession for the unknown soldier arrived between the first, hopeful news, and the last, devastating news about her brother, interpolating a parade line between life and death.

Throughout *The Boys in White* Wheelock was reminded of her brother "at almost every step" (34), in reference to the steps of the funeral procession march during which she first believed, mistakenly, that Orville had been found, and exclaimed her joy "at almost every step" (20). Also in that scene, the women "had gone but a few steps" (20), before they were cut off by the march, thereafter to be utterly disabused of hope. The actual steps of the procession magnified the emotional and obsessional grief that followed, in that each of Wheelock's subsequent footfalls jogged her memory to the dreadful truth about her brother. Her brother's absence contoured Wheelock's narrative, wherein all the dying soldiers she encountered were predeceased by him, and his loss was intensified by all other fatalities. The deaths were legion: as Wheelock mentioned, "Death was a daily visitor" in the hospitals (225). The procession at the beginning became the consuming event, as seen in an alteration in the manuscript, in which Wheelock wrote, "we saw a soldier's funeral approaching" (Ms. 24), then inserted the word "procession" with a caret after "funeral." The addition of "procession" bespoke the leaden rhythm of the march, the dull steps that accompanied the repeated deaths she articulated throughout the memoir. The unending steps of the funeral layered time around her brother's death, giving notice from the beginning that dissolution, inscrutable and open-ended, was always touching the lives of soldiers and nurses.

Wheelock exhibited an internal conflict between using a Christian and secular rhetoric, the first trusting that the dead would find an afterlife, and the second accepting that death was final and earthly. When the news of Orville's death became a reality, Julia Wheelock seemed to believe that her brother would rise again, soothing herself with the Christian promise of resurrection. At other times, her faith became destabilized and her control flagged, so that she expressed a fatalism that excluded faith and evidenced unsettling ideas about the enormity of expiration.[20] Wrestling with Orville's absence at a distance from her family and community, Wheelock mapped a shifting locus of death's significance that never finally consolidated into a single view. Starting nursing work very soon after the news of Orville's passing she met many new patients in the course of her relief work whom she also lost, in turn, to death. Her narrative described a running meditation in which she undertook to understand loss through the discursive filter of Christianity, alternating with a discomfiting pattern of stark realism that at times edged into dread.

The magnetizing phrase "in white" called constant attention most prominently to the hospital's white flag, but carried a myriad of other meanings. For instance, it carried religious overtones, as when Wheelock referenced "a robe of white" in the section containing the unknown soldier's procession: "Father! The pearly gates unfold. . . . And one [angel] has got my starry crown/And one my robe of white" (23). The image in the poem alluded to the Biblical passage: "Who are these, robed in white, and where have they come from?" (Revelation 7:13–14). Because the passage suggests that those "in white" who have suffered never need do so again, it provided solace. Solace of a kind was also suggested when Wheelock nursed a patient, Sergeant Colburn, of Massachusetts, who suffered three severe wounds. She nursed him throughout the night, registered his goodbye look, and the next morning found his body, which she described as "the clay tenement robed in white" (54). Using the touchstone of Revelation she blessed the soldier by reminding the reader that though his body was mortal "clay," he would pass to glory "robed in white."

Still Wheelock, restless in searching for meaning both Christian and secular, suggested that "robed in white" did not always indicate revelatory white robes but sometimes simply the sobering reality that expired soldiers' bodies were at times wrapped in the light-colored blankets of the hospital. It was not unusual for the corpses to remain in the hospital beds for some time before removal, as Wheelock noted: "Graves almost hourly increased in numbers; and even then the demand was not fully met, for it was no uncommon sight to see, in going from tent to tent, from one to half-a-dozen lifeless forms wrapped in their blankets, mutely pleading for burial" (225). Disquietingly, these corpses possessed no robes of glory but only standard-issue hospital bedding. In these cases Wheelock's controlling trope evoked a bleak fatalism, as the deceased patient was covered with nothing but a regulation blanket.

Later in the narrative she amplified the effect of the phrase, "boys in white," to intimate an apparitional rejoinder to the "boys in blue," seeming almost to amass at some times a heavenly, and at other times a ghostly, regiment of the dead. She described the case of another deceased patient who became "enrolled in the army of the 'Boys in White'" (213), and yet another, when she was reunited with Michigan friends who talked and wondered about the absence of mutual acquaintances: "Where were 'Eldred," and 'Birge,' and Woodward?' Had they, too, gone to swell the ranks of the 'Boys in White?'" (43). The phrase operated almost as a refrain whereby Wheelock registered all the new deceased to join in the swelling ranks of white, in the attempt to broach a profound absence.

She oscillated, again, between religion and realism; that is, between reintegrating loss through Christian consolation or coping with loss through a secular and pragmatic, if usually dejected, outlook. When in the latter state, she often leaned toward a dis-integrative mindset that remained in constant recall of Orville. When an awareness of annihilation dictated dejection, she turned and returned to scenes of the funeral procession, which marked the unrenegotiated absence of a loved one. Wheelock experienced unremitting war grief as she wrestled with recurrent successions of decease. Fahs observes that some wartime literature "sought to comprehend and make sense of the violence of war individual by individual, and life by life—a task that grew ever more formidable over the course of the conflict" (119). As Wheelock saw that "the grave was daily closing over 'somebody's darling'" (85), she realized that even language at times failed to frame loss in a way that made sense or offered comfort, as she wished it could for a woman who arrived too late at the bedside of her son. Wheelock reported, "No words of mine could afford her consolation" (148).

At one point, Wheelock visited the U.S. Soldiers's Home, at the grounds of which "thousands of the 'boys in white' lie buried, and their number is daily increasing" (169). From Wheelock's point of view of incessant carnage the graves represented "many a broken home circle" (169), a brokenness expressing her own family's loss as well. She underscored the countless numbers gone: "Thither have been brought thousands of the suffering 'boys in blue,' and from them have been removed multitudes of lifeless 'boys in white'" (170). One of the major characteristics of the female nurse's experience, differentiated to some degree from even the soldier's experience, was the ceaseless occurrence of death in the hospital; the soldier of course saw horrible suffering and death in the field, but also underwent days of marching, camping, and waiting, sometimes for weeks at a time, while the nurse, especially if working during the last years of the war, seldom escaped a day of loss among the rows of men under her charge. The Civil War nurse who attempted to make sense of death found the problem compounded by the fact that she faced it daily, in tides of incoming casualties, and used coping behaviors that were exceptionally complicated, moment-based, and recurring.

Probably the most dejected moment in *The Boys in White* occurred after the Battle of Fredericksburg, as Wheelock and other workers waited for the wounded to arrive. She reported fatalities with a sense that the war lacked purpose altogether: "Our loss is estimated at ten thousand—another great slaughter and nothing gained" (69). She betrayed a tone of sorrow without recourse to reason, and then added further this brief and memorable comment: "Oh! When will these scenes of carnage cease? Echo answers, 'when!'" (69). The terse sentence—"Echo answers, 'when!'"—suggested an existential dialogue with an echo, obviating human interaction altogether. Frighteningly, the only word left was the resounding "when!"—spoken by no one. This iteration indicated perpetuity, precluding redemption, and repeating itself, the note of "when!" sounding without resolution.

Two concrete scenes exemplify the fact that Wheelock moved alternately between consolation and dejection as they occurred side-by-side throughout *The Boys in White*. Both responses took place during her visit to the site of the Battle of Chantilly, where Orville was fatally wounded. Wheelock responded to grief during the Chantilly scenes by shifting from a state of dread that was secular and bleak, to a state of reintegration that was religious and elegiac. The two scenes revealed first dread, when she visited the battlefield, and second reintegration, when she visited the Chantilly farm a few days later; this second, reintegrative mourning was grounded in Christian faith but also in abolitionist rhetoric.

Visiting the site of the Battle of Chantilly, Wheelock reconstructed a vivid scenario of her brother's suffering: "upon this very field he fell; here for days he lay beneath the scorching rays of a Southern sun, torn and mangled, bleeding, dying—no hope of ever again seeing home or wife or child" (96). Her imaginings didn't stop at personal grief: "Then multiply his case by thousands, and oh, what a scene was here witnessed!" (96). As she relived her brother's death, her lament for him amplified into a lament for many, the reality enlarging to include "thousands." She witnessed the Chantilly landscape markers: the ball-pierced tree, the shattered buildings, the ravaged tree branches, the exploded earth, some human bones "protruding" (97), some skulls slightly exposed. Her grim observations obviated the chance for the relative comfort of mourning, and her suggestion that her brother's fate had been multiplied in the fates of many other boys in white attested to a grief still active.

By contrast, a few days later she rode back to the site, but stopped instead at Chantilly farm, a property of several hundred acres that was "lovely, even in its desolation" (99). She surveyed the property that lacked the original fences but still showcased a carriageway "with shade-trees upon either side" (99), the grounds graced with shrubs and evergreens. In an even more comely area at the back of the mansion, Wheelock realized that Chantilly farm was not abandoned after all, for she met an elderly black couple who "were living there in a small cabin, probably their former quarters" (100). Wheelock attempted, like Holstein, to seize the terms of abolitionism to lift her flagging sense of the war's meaning, as she reported the elderly man saying, "'we'se allus slaves till Massa Lincoln free us'" (100). The man reckoned himself to be about 100 years old, a life span that indicated his birth predated the Revolutionary War, which marked American independence from England, to the present moment of the Civil War, which marked independence for the slave. Wheelock seemed to suggest that in light of the emancipation enjoyed by these two African American elders, the loss of life experienced by soldiers and the grief experienced by survivors had warrant. The moment, however, was in part marred by the fact Wheelock used a stock, sentimental scene common in many nineteenth-century fictional works. Wheelock, politically adept at using the rhetoric of antislavery, exhibited the same bias as other white nurses in presenting a black human being as a conceptual marker to aid her ideological goals, and in this scene employed the couple as a stand-in for a reprieve in her own grief, as an unfortunate metaphor for the hope that loss would be mitigated.

Wheelock continued to struggle with ways to absorb her experience of grief throughout *The Boys in White*. Often, the fact of demise possessed its own peremptory momentum and landscape, as Wheelock attested: "Death is at work, the lone ambulance on its way to the 'silent city' too plainly tells" (66). Throughout the war years she worked in unresolved bereavement, describing, for example, in a way reminiscent of Holstein, a patient dying of typhoid fever, who "lingered long weeks on the narrow space which separated the 'now from the hereafter'" (127–28).[21] Alternately consoled and dejected, Wheelock again attempted, at the end of her memoir, to cope with the alternation of states of grief.

First, moving toward consolation, she embraced in the terms of Abraham Lincoln's death, a patriotic wholeness, and second, moving toward dejection, she revisited in her imagination the empty hospitals that seemed to hold the unsettled spirits of expired soldiers. Wheelock, along with millions of Americans, mourned the death of Lincoln, and looked for wartime closure by focusing intensively on the obsequies. She had the "sad privilege to see the remains of our lamented President" twice, viewing his body at the Capitol and the White House (255). Emblems of mourning were everywhere visible at this time, especially in "that long procession"—a movement with a multitude of boys in blue, including "infantry, cavalry, and artillery, with various bands; the Marine Corps and band; officers of the army and navy; Congressmen; members of the Cabinet, the Diplomatic Corps," and more (255).[22] The capital witnessed the grand funeral review, a review that probably caused Wheelock to recall the funeral procession of the unknown soldier she'd witnessed at the outset of the narrative, before she'd been informed of Orville's death and after which she searched continually for condolence. This time using patriotic discourse, Wheelock presented the grand review as if Lincoln's death might redeem the deaths of all soldiers, and through this she seemed to find partial relief. In the country's procession for the slain president, she momentarily reset grief toward condolence and was granted a moment of mourning.

Juxtaposed with Wheelock's witnessing of the grand review was her passing of the hospitals where she'd worked before preparing to leave Washington, DC to return home. She remembered in detail the soldiers at these hospitals who had suffered and expired. With this revisiting she shaped her narrative, finally, into a consideration of the nature of memory: "I can never efface from memory the feelings of loneliness experienced in passing through those empty hospitals. Each ward seemed like a haunted house, where the spirits of the departed still lingered" (260–61). The spirits, habitual, haunted her slightly, so that she was troubled by an inability fully to absorb a reintegrative kind of mourning. The venture of Wheelock's narrative turned on her response to death, which at this turn in the book tended toward the ghostly. She despaired about those patients' lives that remained unreclaimable, recalling case after case of suffering that she "might continue to enumerate" but, she added, "the memory of them is too painful" (262).

Probably every war narrative is at heart a consideration of the nature of memory, concerned with the stakes of internalizing wrenching experience. Many war narratives close with a mixture of desolation and hope, and Wheelock's, too, circumvented any comfortable presentation of loss by declining to register memory as either compensatory or fracturing. She refused to fix an attitude toward that first funeral procession, and remained at a crossroads in the end: "In retrospecting the past, I find conflicting emotions alternately taking possession of my heart, emotions both of joy and sorrow" (265). Her conflict spoke to an experience in which no single form of bereavement took precedence, and the experience of loss continued to recur. In the final pages of Wheelock's narrative, she attempted to fulfill the expectations of her culture by renouncing dread and embracing comfort, but she could not completely fuse her past war experiences with her postwar present. The fact that *The Boys in White*, published in 1870, was the last nurse narrative written for a decade highlights its difficult status in delivering an elegiac message when the war was finished but the memories were still raw. Though Wheelock did live a full life in the years after the war, marrying and having children, at the endpoint of her narrative she confided that, "the sad reflections far outweigh all the pleasant experiences" (265).[23]

In this, Wheelock refused to placate her audience with sentimental patriotism and Christianity, lamenting that it was "sad to see so many crippled youth, so many empty sleeves" (266), and continuing to think, concerning the multitudes of dead, that "the price seems too costly" (266). This was the last sentence of the narrative that carried gravitas, though she wrote four more sentences,[24] followed by a quotation from Lincoln and consolation poetry written by others, which occupied six pages; this end matter seemed to speak, as did the last pages of Holstein, to sentiments of reconciliation and commemoration that were not her own. That she resorted to such extensive citation in the final pages possibly indicated a reluctance or inability to articulate her opinions in her own words. In fact, the tacked-on conclusion did not actually exist in her manuscript, for the book's citations of consolatory materials were added at a later date. In considering the tone of the narrative as a whole, the brief sentence interrogating suffering, spoken much earlier in the narrative, carried the greater weight: "Echo answers, 'when!'" This tone of near-nihilistic abandon, derived from the positing of a world that functioned to efface survivors—save for the retainer of a mocking "when!"—is one of the sad, possibly subliminal, but undeniable powers behind Julia Wheelock's *The Boys in White*.

Our work was among every class of men who wore the uniforms of soldiers, and they represented almost every household in the land. They were the bone and sinew of the country....—Sophronia Bucklin (34)

CONCLUSION

To a reading public, the woman nurse came to typify a national character to be appreciated along with the profusion of national characters portrayed in nineteenth-century texts. The nurse narrator inscribed herself as representative of the woman nurse who worked in the hospital or camp and maneuvered through the difficulties of the new job. She was a fresh type of the American who underwent traumas of privation and illness as a part of the work, her trials coterminous with those of the nation. As she shaped her identity, so did the country; that is to say, the American narrative in general was crucial to national character at any given time in the history of the country, as Sharon Harris asserts, for example, of the decades of 1790 through 1830: "The writing and reading of historical narratives was considered essential in the construction of an 'American' identity, as the ancient and recent pasts became the interpretive field upon which the integrity of the new nation would be built" (Introduction vii). The narrative a few decades later, in the time span of 1863–70, was at least as important in offering an interpretive field upon which to build national identity.

A tactful yet persistent chronicler of the war, the narrator depicted the nurse as an exemplar of efficiency and professionalism, savior of the soldier, and prospective model of the new woman.[1] The nurse memoirist proclaimed her investment in the American working class, heralding the common soldier as the real war hero and speaking purposefully to affirm his natural heroism. Inverting the conventional social order, she supported the rank-and-file to praise acts of duty over pedigrees of status. In creating countless quick-stroke verbal portraits of army privates, she praised all working Americans, and in crafting scenes to prove the common man's native decency she testified to the country's fortitude and resilience. At a time when Americans were reconceiving ideas of female subjectivity and community, those concepts were contoured by the presence of women within the hospital workplace—a place that was often raw and sometimes hostile but that afforded women the chance to test their abilities.

The woman relief worker owned a front seat at the disassembling and incipient rebuilding of the country, describing from that vantage an in-process and continually redelineated democracy. She acted as both champion and interlocutor of the American republic, which stood as a national experiment not even a century old, a republic that during the Civil War was in danger of disintegrating. The nurse readjusted conceptions of medical care to fit the rough actuality of understaffed, underequipped wards housing men with debilitating illnesses; additionally, she tested her response to social and political issues in flux as she lived them in the hospital, retooling the rhetoric of women's rights and abolitionism to shape new understandings of the project of egalitarian nation-making. The hospital located a gripping workshop, so to speak, on United States democracy-in-operation during a time of aggravated change, when social ideologies were thrown into high relief.

For the citizen of the era, navigating the complicated terrain of gender, class, race, and ethnicity was almost unavoidable. The nurse narrator took out her pencil and made notes on these complications, fashioning them into a memoir for an audience invested in wartime difficulties. She and other nurses crossed social lines to establish camaraderie with patients and workers from different demographics, including black, Native American, and immigrant populations. David Blight asserts that the American sensibility was remade by a diverse group of laborers, including the "thousands of surviving soldiers, liberated freedpeople enduring near starvation in contraband camps, and women on both homefronts who performed all manner of war work and tried to sustain farms, households, and the human spirit as their men were asked to die for ideas, self-defense, retribution, manly values, or some abstract notion of their community's future" (18). The nurse narrator chronicled her interactions with diverse groups at the hospitals and camps, these interactions part of the brace of mutual acknowledgement needed to rebuild the country. The hospital itself served as a new model of United States democracy, a locale into which the nurse ventured daily.[2] She lived at the forefront of the shifting contours of social order, where people of various demographics regularly came into contact in encounters previously untried on such a scale. While the hospital posed challenges because of social disparities, it also housed people of different origins, and their proximity at times exemplified possible democratic affinities. The body politic was represented by the ward, the hospital, or the camp itself.

Mapping a progression in the rhetoric used by nurse narrators during the period can be a difficult business, given that this project examines seven texts over eight years, making the discernment of definitive patterns a narrow endeavor; nonetheless, a few impressions take hold in reading these memoirs in succession. First, we have seen the nurse narrator building a strong conversational apparatus to win over her audience —for instance, Alcott's question-and-answer, Woolsey's direct pleas for supplies, Dunlap's use of a persona to stand in for the reader—and then we have seen the conversational apparatus continuing in a strong but not so tightly controlled way. The tone of conversation remained and was always dependent on narratorial performance, but eased into a comfortable repartee that was more often tacit than structurally imposed. Powers' smart volubility, for instance, or Bucklin's lengthy accounts of confrontations with officials attested to an understood bond with readers, a continual and informal conversational women's rhetoric the memoirists nurtured through their works.

In addition, the nurse's discourse of racial accord, often a profession of accord that did not match her actions, was more or less a constant throughout the narratives. If, previous to the Proclamation, the nurse had been animated by antislavery discourse and the promise of liberty for all races, she afterward became unreliably or only intermittently committed to advocating for racial parity. At best, nurse narrators moved from the rhetoric of freedom to a clumsy articulation of social equality and unity. The nurse narratives did, nonetheless, evidence a progress from the mixed abolitionist rhetoric of Alcott and Woolsey in 1863 to the more honest personal observations of Bucklin in 1869, demonstrating an uneven trajectory in increased awareness of white hypocrisy. Toni Morrison's stipulation, quoted in the introduction, that the "Africanist presence" is ubiquitous in American literature, can be proved on most of these narratives, given especially Morrison's interest, again, in "what prompts and makes possible this process of entering what one is estranged from . . . into corners of the consciousness held off and away from the reach of the writer's imagination" (4). Exactly this condition of estrangement held away in corners of white consciousness inhered in the nurse memoirs, the consciousness increasing toward partial enlightenment in the later memoirs.

We also have seen an increase in three different rhetorical trends. Clearly, the nurse memoirs evidenced more dissent in the later texts than the earlier, as Schultz and other scholars have pointed out. Not surprisingly, a strong reliance on the rhetoric of women's rights accompanied this rise in dissent, Powers, and Bucklin especially drawing authority from the rhetoric to counter the effects of negligence and graft. At the same time, they tracked the lines of gendered communication in the workplace in order to attempt to find a powerful position from which a woman could speak from within her job.

In addition, we've seen an increase in the interrogation of suffering as a corrective for the nation. This interrogation was always relatively scarce, and in most cases muted, but it showed slightly with Powers's work, then formed a bit more fully in the works of Holstein and Wheelock. Despite its rarity, the interrogation of suffering may have been one of the most valuable of the nurse narrator contributions. As the nurse advocated for diverse hospital patients, she interrogated the suffering of war. Her stance of patriotic loyalty to country remained one of surprising complexity, given its centrality to her project. Most Northern women, of course, robustly espoused the cause of the Union, bespeaking loyalty to country as demonstrated by their service, but some used a different tenor to animate their allegiance, as they quietly inquired into the problem of assigning meaning to suffering. Powers asked about a misdiagnosed patient with the question, "He has fallen a victim to what?" (171); Holstein was undone by the need to express the physical agony of the "perfect skeleton" of a living man returning from Andersonville (127); and Wheelock contemplated the senselessness of war in the words, "Echo answers, 'When!'" (69). The moments during which pain subsumed the text revealed the crux at which articulation proved the most visceral, scrappy, and unprocessed. The women discovered at some points that words of consolation carried no power in the face of the body's defilement.[3]

Finally, concerning the American character, the nurse attended to patients, but the nurse narrator attended to an audience by creating a first-person speaker and main character worthy of her era.[4] Possessing a unique position from which to chronicle the war, she observed a country at cross-purposes and faced the problem in personal and familial ways. Bent on establishing a conversational bond with her readers, she confided in them with the assuring tone of an ally who, like the women at home, was the primary healer in the family circle, a circle that now extended to the country. Schultz observes that the tumult of the 1860s jarred the expected order of things and admitted of social restructuring: "A social order in transition—in this case brought about by war—is one in which both new sexual and textual paradigms may emerge" ("Performing Genres" 80). One of the most prominent of such new sexual and textual paradigms surfaced in the form of the narrative that allowed the nurse to integrate fresh experiences into women's accomplishments and thereby stake a claim to the importance of a new female American character.

Elizabeth Cady Stanton wrote near the end of the nineteenth century that "the achievements of women" in the Civil War have been left untold in that they "do not figure in the official reports" and that "the names of thousands are unknown beyond the neighborhood where they lived or the hospitals where they loved to labor" (235). Stanton's point is well-taken; many women who labored in the war were omitted from the official record and thousands remain unknown. The nurse memoirist of the 1860s began the work of representing those thousands and registering women's achievements in the personal, distinctive voice of the popular literature of the time. Sizer reminds us that, "in moments of national definition, trauma, and change, the power of the teller increases exponentially" (6). The nurse memoirist may have guessed at the increased power of the teller, the native value of owning a story in that agitated time, and the probability of cultivating sympathetic readers.

The narrator examined and gauged national values, and emerged after the war with a distinct identity as a representative woman, perhaps partially in answer to the *Representative Men* of Ralph Waldo Emerson, who in 1856 asserted that certain people are lenses on the world, "lenses through which we read our own minds," and that we seek the "*otherest*" people as our greatest and most cherished models (*Representative Men* 11, 12). The Civil War nurse is a serious contender for an "otherest" person, as she overcame early perceptions of women nurses as nuisances, distractions, and obstructionists. Against adverse publicity, the narrator emphasized the character of nurse service, adhering to the presentation of feminine moral probity as she wrote a personal history that expressed the raw quandaries of her new, untried, "otherest" service to country. She tendered a timely cultural alternative in presenting the female nurse as "representative" of a gendered patriotic personality.

To come full circle in this study, we can recall that Alcott's character, Tribulation Periwinkle, was advised by her family on the first page of *Hospital Sketches* that of the several options open to women for "something to do," the first option was that she could write a book. Though she chose to attend to soldiers, choosing to write a book, it turned out, was imbedded in the experience for Alcott, who seized the challenges of being both nurse and narrator because she saw these dual achievements as vital to her sense of self and her duty to country. She initiated, as did the other women nurses studied here, a fresh form of address—an instigative type of war literature prominent for telling, at crucial impasses, clean-edged truths. The nurse memoir became a small arena in which the American woman tested a new national identity, attempting to make sense, in a rugged workplace, of both devastating and at times miraculous contingencies for the republic. Inviting the reader into the process of identity creation as an essential factor in the process, the nurse narrator cared for soldiers and duly inscribed that care to actualize a female national character.

NOTES

Introduction

1. For each nurse narrator, the citation refers to her nurse narrative, unless otherwise indicated.

2. From the totality of the twelve narratives, I have exempted five: Katharine Wormeley's 1863 *United States Sanitary Commission*, Sarah Emma Edmonds's 1865 *Nurse and Spy in the Union Army*, Jane Hoge's 1867 *Boys in Blue*, Jane Stuart Woolsey's 1868 *Hospital Days*, and Sarah Palmer's 1867 *The Story of Aunt Becky's Army-Life*. I exclude the Wormeley, Edmonds, Hoge, and Jane Woolsey mainly because they do not to a great degree own the particular qualities of the personal memoir. The thrust of Wormeley's book is to present a history of the Sanitary Commission, replete with statistics, inspectors' duties, addresses, and various reports. Edmonds' bestselling book portrays some nursing activities, but differs materially in its presentation of audacious adventures, many undoubtedly romanticized. Hoge's voluminous book is historical, about nursing, but also a compendium of other war experiences, the chapters including the actions of relief organizations, military logistics, sketches of well-known personalities, and also chapters written by others, such as Mary Livermore; it "less often reflected the fictionalized coming-of-age narrative" (Schultz 223). Jane Woolsey's text has many of the qualities of the personal memoir, but from the perspective of a hospital administrator, and with the partial objective to organize the facility and argue for the training of women nurses; also, because I have chosen to examine the work of her sister Georgeanna Woolsey, I release Jane Stuart Woolsey's narrative so as to represent narrators from diverse backgrounds and areas of the country. Sarah Palmer's case is different; I am dissuaded from analyzing her fascinating text for the narratological reason that the book was "written by her niece, Sylvia Lawson Covey, and based on interviews with Palmer and her diary of three months" (Sizer 211), qualities that counteract the single-author stipulation for this study and curtail the ability to study it as a constructed narrative written for the purpose of an individual narrator engaging with an audience.

3. Woolsey's narrative covers only Gettysburg, but she went on to work at other sites throughout the war.

4. Jane Schultz's groundbreaking history, *Women at the Front*, examines the work of a large number of Northern and Southern nurses, both during and after the war, and stands as a necessary precursor to any study of Civil War nurse narratives. By contrast, my study intensively examines the experiences of only seven nurses during a discrete period of eight years and focuses on the strategies by which the nurses expressed their experiences in written narratives. Every Schultz citation refers to her book, *Women at the Front*, unless otherwise noted.

5. Here, as everywhere in this book, the italicized emphasis is not mine, and is always that of the quoted author, unless otherwise indicated.

6. Male convalescent nurses were seen as the social equivalent of the charity case or almshouse resident. In the public's mind, patients in civilian hospitals "had to rely on aged inmates, prisoners, derelects [*sic*] or, at best, down-and-outs who could not find a job doing anything else." Nursing hardly presented itself as a viable work option, let alone a job for middle-class women—"certainly no *lady*" was a nurse (Brooks 52). The relatively few women nurses in civilian hospitals before the war were, like the male nurses, largely destitute and transient. It was rare for middle-class women to work in a hospital institution before mid-century. People of most classes were nursed at home, and only the "deserving poor" used hospitals, staffed by untrained nurses more or less "indistinguishable from housemaids" (Bostridge 95).

7. Nightingale's work made her famous in England, where she was celebrated "in terms reserved for living Saints" (Penner xii). In January 1861, the *Godey's Lady's Book* cover featured five women "depicted as ideals on pedestals" (Okker 116), the most prominent among them Nightingale and Dorothea Dix, the crusader for the rights of the mentally ill, who became Superintendent of Women Nurses for the Union forces in June 1861. The figures were flanked by six scenes of women engaged in service work that "made the phenomenon of women in the workplace visible and nameable" (Tonkovich 62). An accompanying essay urged women to undertake nursing outside the home. The issue easily reached tens of thousands of readers: *Godey*'s circulation in 1861 was 150,000 (by contrast, *Harper's New Monthly Magazine* was 110,00 at about the same time, *Atlantic Monthly*'s less than 50,000 during its highest point) (Bennett 231). The Nightingale example pervaded mid-nineteenth-century American culture to the point that later a *New York Herald* editorial headlined in 1864, "'All Our Women Are Florence Nightingales'" (quoted in Reverby 44).

8. Nightingale's example also bolstered the nurses who succeeded her, because she wrote about the work, for example in her most famous book, *Notes on Nursing: What It Is and What It Is Not*. The English edition appeared in 1859, the American edition in 1860, a slim volume arriving on the cusp of war to inspire female relief workers. The book sold "15,000 copies within two months" and, not

surprisingly, *Godey's* urged "every lady" to study it (Bostridge 357, 361). Instructing every place of healing to prize cleanliness, character, training, organization, and moral backbone, Nightingale's book offered a crisp, almost tart rhetoric. It is easy to imagine that an aspiring nurse narrator would have been riveted by prose that, as Dunbar states, possessed "'a clearness not unmixed with notes of humorous sub-acidity'" (xvii). Nightingale proved so certain of women's powers of healing that she argued that accidents (such as suicide, bleeding to death, and other cases of neglect) happened in hospitals under men's watch, and "would not" happen under a woman's (40).

9. Schultz finds that of the forty-three published monographs written by women in the decades during and after the war, about three times as many were written by Union women (thirty-two as opposed to twelve) (220).

10. One of the exceptions is Walt Whitman's 1875 *Memoranda During the War*, a memoir of nursing experience traditionally more famous and critically acknowledged than the narratives studied here, though theirs predate his. Indeed, Whitman's text has in decades past been tacitly and inaccurately assumed to stand as the primary example of Civil War nurse narrative; in fact he most likely modeled his work on these earlier narratives.

11. Alice Fahs describes the lack of war literature publications in general during the 1870s, noting that *Harper's Weekly*, "which had published well over one hundred Civil War stories during and immediately after the war . . . published only two Civil War stories during the entire decade of the 1870s" (313). For financial reasons, the publication industry after the war may have shepherded authors toward new material. Michael Gilmore, for example, suggests that after such a cataclysmic rupture the country distrusted the textual work of narrative itself: "Bloodletting on such a vast scale discredited words in two ways: it made them seem insignificant beside the numberless dead, and it pronounced them culpable for the carnage in the first place" (9). Schultz suggests the reason for the gap may have been that women nurses after the war turned their attention to organizing educational opportunities for future nurses, setting up soldier welfare relief, and teaching in schools for freedpeople, and that after the 1870s dearth "the market improved in the 1880s" (310).

12. I happened to discover independently that the author's name was Julia Dunlap before finding the information in an unassuming footnote in Schultz's 2010 edited volume, *This Birthplace of Souls*.

13. Silber asserts that while many historians have read the Civil War as a "prod to feminism," she would "caution against reading the Civil War as a moment of female liberation" (*Daughters* 10, 11). The mid-century years offered a range of civic activities for Northern women to strengthen their voices in the cause of the Union, but did not provide opportunities specifically for women's rights.

Wendy Hamand Venet states the priorities of women activists shifted around mid-century: "Although many female abolitionists regarded woman's rights as their first priority after 1848, this order was reversed with the outbreak of war" (18). Venet asserts that, "woman's rights conventions that had taken place annually in the 1850s ceased" (18).

14. Though examining writing after the war, Sicherman observes a pattern that could describe the war period as well: "The scarcity of models of nontraditional womanhood has prompted women more often than men to turn to literature for self-authorization" (*Well-Read Lives* 2).

15. The works in this study fall on the cusp between sentimentality and realism. I don't pursue that observation, because nurse narratives are not works of fiction, which usually provide the subject matter for the larger scholarly conversation about sentimentality and realism. The nurse narrative occupies the porous space between the two movements as, for instance, Harris has shown of Rebecca Harding Davis's "Life in the Iron Mills," which blended styles of moralistic outlook and reformist impulse, showing the everyday "commonplace [so as] to expose the harsh realities of life" (Davis 11). All seven narratives contain both sentimental and realist features. Dunlap, for instance, draws prominently on sentimental fiction, specifically referencing Harriet Beecher Stowe's "right feeling," a hallmark of sentimentality and moral suasion in antebellum fiction. The memoirs also draw at times on realist fiction, notably Holstein's work, which progresses almost to a bleak naturalism at the end. The nurses' realism could also be considered in light of Andrew Lawson's recent work, which treats realism in terms of the downwardly mobile, those who suffer most from a "radically destabilized social structure" (4). Poignantly, Lawson sees this set of questions as determining the outlook of realism: "Can I trust the world to look the same tomorrow as it does today? Do the things I own have any stable or enduring value?" (2). In varying degrees, every nurse narrator posed these questions during the Civil War.

16. Unfortunately, this study does not cover works written after 1870 and so does not analyze the insightful nurse narrative of the African American nurse, Susie King Taylor, who wrote the 1902 *Reminiscences of My Life in Camp*.

17. Arac uses "narrative" to apply to both fiction and nonfiction.

18. They were conditioned by reading the eighteenth-century sentimental novel, including the Bildungsroman, and the autobiography, including notably Benjamin Franklin's; they constructed their own lives by featuring themselves as "author-protagonists" (Casper 14).

19. Mattingly identifies temperance advocates as "the largest group of women orators" in the nineteenth century. They showed "an exceptional understanding of language use within the cultural context of their time" (Mattingly 1); she

observes that the temperance movement included both progressive and conservative elements.

20. Mattingly discusses the need for temperance speakers to develop "rhetorical skills in a manner 'appropriate' to and successful for their gender" (7), and Bacon discusses the rhetorical tactic of discussing "an 'unfeminine' topic while professing to avoid it" (161). Women of both movements dealt with topics both "delicate" and "indelicate," as Childs notes about Harriet Jacobs's difficult narrative task, for instance, of slave women having to speak about rape.

21. Partly because popular opinion was so divided about female relief workers, Superintendent of Nurses Dorothea Dix set stringent requirements for Civil War women nurses, including the stipulations that women nurses be at least thirty years of age and have a matronly appearance. It is no wonder that women turned to boosting their maternal characteristics to defend their character, given Dix's requirements for service: women "sober, earnest, self-sacrificing, and self-sustained; who can bear the presence of suffering and exercise entire self-control, of speech and manner; who can be calm, gentle, quiet, active, and steadfast in duty, also who are willing to take and to execute the directions of the surgeons of the divisions in which they are stationed" (Brown 283). Only paragons of virtue and temperament were expected to apply.

22. Some nurse narrators made ingenious use of a first-person anonymous voice to refine authorial power, defer narrative identity, and comment more freely on prevailing cultural factors. The works of Woolsey, Dunlap, and Holstein made use of such discontinuities, each employing occluded forms of address to protect her social standing or slyly to counter negative societal perceptions of nurse viability.

23. Delafield notes that, "the diary presents the unmediated reflection of a life without interpretation whilst autobiography overwrites a life already lived with knowledge of narrative closure" (15). Nurse narratives, while not polished autobiographies, moved at least a half-step away from diary entries toward civic expression.

24. Again, Whitman, in his fragmented *Memoranda*, has been credited with anticipating contemporary wartime journalism (such as journalists' on-the-pulse accounts of Vietnam in the twentieth century), but the narratives examined here preceded his by some years.

25. The aesthetic of immediacy appeared in several compositional ways: grammatical inflections, lack of transitions, and use of the dash. Some grammatical inflections, for example, included the use of incomplete sentences. For instance, Powers used the informal gesture of omitting the sentence subject, "I," as she wrote in the rush of her new assignment to a smallpox hospital. Holstein's work at times lacked paragraph transitions, her prose pivoting from idea

to idea and scene to scene as she chronicled traumatic, disjunctive scenes. Some nurses peppered diction with dashes, a stylistic flourish used often in the nineteenth century for personal writings but usually dropped for more formal work. In some nurse narratives, writers retained the dash to indicate that the transition from informal to formal expression, or from private to national address, was hurried or incomplete.

26. Only Holstein can be verified as married at the time; Alcott, Woolsey, Bucklin, and Wheelock can be verified as single. Dunlap and Powers never mention a husband. Though unmarried status does not prove that the nurse had no children, of course, it suggests the unlikelihood of the nurse having children, especially as all but one of these nurses left home to serve, and so would have had to set up childcare in their absence.

27. Sizer points out that "class issues took on new relevance for middle-class women concerned about national unity as well as eager to establish a vision of universal womanhood" (8).

28. By decomposition I also mean *de-composition*, the process of writing the undoing enacted by death and the bald fact of decay and putrefaction. I mean, too, the articulation of words that unmake themselves, that undo inscription in the face of an event that lacked words to match the enormity of experience. I mean disarticulation, an unleashing of the presumed strands of the purport attached to an experience that suddenly become unavailable to linguistic maneuvers, and certainly unavailable to patriotism.

Chapter One

1. They appeared in *The Commonwealth* on May 22, May 29, June 12, and June 26 of 1863, and would be modified for the book's chapters, "A Day," "A Night," "Off Duty," and "A Postscript."

2. I note here the lack of apostrophe in "don't" with "[*sic*]," but will refrain from noting other such characteristic anomalies (with the exception of unusual spellings that I want to make sure are not mistaken for typographical errors).

3. Fahs mentions this to suggest "the possibility that soldiers' own views of their hospital experiences may have been shaped by wartime popular literature" (115).

4. Young argues, too, that Alcott affiliates her female nurse experience with the wounded male soldier experience, a move by which "her illness gains new value, constructed as a soldier's battle service," and thus "grants new narrative power" (83). Both Young's book and this one are concerned with narrative power, the former in a gendered argument that sees Alcott masculinizing Trib-

ulation's experience, and this one with a gendered argument that sees Alcott directly addressing and placating her audience to gain maximal reception.

5. Though literary historians often use the present tense in writing about literary works, the past tense is employed in this book as the least distracting way to read about these hybrid texts (like *Hospital Sketches*, for example).

6. In these chapters Alcott introduced the elements of motivation and travel that would become staples in the narratives that followed hers; Sarah Emma Edmonds's narrative, though not examined here, showed direct emulation and cribbing of phrases from Alcott; Dunlap and Holstein may have alluded to Alcott, as mentioned in the chapters on each; Wheelock marked an Alcott poem in her scrapbook.

7. The suggestion of acting on a stage was a dicey proposition, risking social reproach for the actress. The suggestions reveal the meager choices available to women of the time.

8. We would expect that the family of Louisa May Alcott would have responded to her decision to go nurse the soldiers with enthusiasm and idealism, especially given that the family was presided over by the ebullient Bronson Alcott; no wonder Tribulation's family built a utopian hospital in their minds. At different moments owning and rejecting her family's eccentricities, Alcott oscillated in her opinion of them. Once, she contacted Redpath about hastening the publication of one of her works so that she could have money to support her family: "He [Redpath] sent it to the printers at once so there was another little help for this incapable family"; later, she "canceled 'incapable' and inserted 'rising'" (*Journals* 121,125).

9. Her phrase, "aerial architecture," recalls the advice of fellow Concord native Henry David Thoreau: "If you have built castles in the air, your work need not be lost; that is where they should be. Now put the foundations under them" (563).

10. Scholars such as Giesberg, Silber, and Sizer have posited nurses' mediation between homefront and warfront.

11. The scene of the matron subtly recalls Tribulation's leaving home, relying on the centering image of her own mother, "the memory of the dear old lady," which imparted strength and purpose to scenes of upheaval.

12. The matron in question was Hannah Ropes, whose letters, generally unavailable until 1980, record her resistance to hospital injustice based on her authority as mother. In one contretemps with a superior, Ropes states that she would take on the conflict all over again: "Why? Because I am a mother, and I have only to remember that each of these sick ones [has] a mother somewhere, and for the time I act for them" (89).

13. This cover was unlike the insignia on other Redpath publications from 1863, which displayed a pine or palm tree ensconced in an ornate oval with a necklace-like string along the bottom.

14. Alcott must have relied on her memory for the words, because the short clause does not appear in Dickens in that exact form, although Sarah Gamp says she wishes to give "no offence" several times in the novel. The epigraph seemed to arise as an amalgamation of two different speakers from the novel, Mrs. Sarah Gamp and George Chuzzlewit. Gamp comes closest when she says, "'Which no offence is meant, ladies and gentlemen; none bein' took, I hope'" (526). George Chuzzlewit utters the "naming no names" phrase (46).

15. This criticism was more pointed in the book than in the newspaper columns.

16. Promising in effect not to point a finger at any particular personage, she kept her promise, in her book though not her journal, in which she did specify actual people. Alcott stipulated that she kept her journal only for herself and no one else, and so identified many of the people with whom she worked: "My society consists of Miss Kendal, Miss [Lizzie] Thurber, Mrs Ropes, Mrs Cramer, my room mate, & a few very disagreeable women whom I dont care to know. Drs Otman, Fitz Patrick, Hyde, Smith & Winslow are the gentleman [*sic*]" (115). In the *Sketches* she designated the doctors only by the initials, Dr. O., Dr. P., and Dr. Z.

17. Payn points out in an 1880 article on narrative that authors used blanks for names because they feared being charged with "actions of libel" (316).

18. Interestingly, she changed a nurse's name, "Miss Faithful," in *The Commonwealth* newspaper version, to "Miss Blank" (62) in the book.

19. The encomiums were renewed when the 1869 version of *Hospital Sketches* was issued, one commenter, for example, praising the book as being "full of bright touches" (*Zion's Herald* Sept 2, 1869). Most readers saw not only the bright touches but the difficult aspects of hospital life as well, the "graphic pictures" (*Harper's* Nov 1869)—what Alcott would have called "the dismals."

20. I return to "A Postscript" as it appeared in the book, and distinguish it from the same segment appearing as an installment in *The Commonwealth*. In the book chapter, Alcott enlarged upon instances of severity as a way, possibly, to counter the complaint of that "serious-minded party who objected to a tone of levity." She had been describing several comic hospital incidents, then added a two-page segment possibly for the purposes of self-correction: "This is the comic side of the matter. The serious one is harder to describe" (65). After writing this she recalled several deathbed scenes that were particularly wrenching—a father tending a dying son, a wife finding that her husband had died, and

a sister whose brother had passed away before she arrived to say her farewell. Tribulation's reaction to this sister was unguarded: "So, feeling heart-sick, home-sick, and not knowing what else to do, I just put my arms about her, and began to cry in a very helpless but hearty way" (67).

21. Alcott also expanded the book chapter in other significant ways, including dissenting opinions: a paragraph on a chaplain who, though claiming he had no Secessionist leanings, nonetheless "seceded from his ministerial duties (63), and a new segment on the heedless Dr. P, whose manner was so insensitive that Alcott wished to use his own "disagreeable," sharp instruments on him" (71). (The portrait of Dr. P, however, was offset with that of Dr. Z, a doctor of great warmth and kindness; Alcott seemed always to be balancing these things.) The expansion in the book served as a sort of remedy to the reader's complaint that her columns lacked gravitas.

22. Twice having imagined chaos and death, Tribulation finally fell asleep on the boat, and when she did, dreamed "of muffins" (15)—clearly a joke by which Alcott recovered her character's cheer, offering a commonplace, banal image to counterpoise the waking dreams of destruction.

23. Raised by a Transcendental family that nurtured sanguine views, she was conditioned to see the bright side, but paid a price for it when bleak visions appeared.

24. Freud defines the "*Heimliche*" as belonging to the "house or family" (222) and the "*Unheimliche*" (or uncanny) as the "un-home-y" material that recurs in a frightening or unfamiliar way.

25. Although she was anxious about how her audience might receive her views, Alcott was unapologetic about her fervid abolitionist loyalties, publishing part of the material in *The Commonwealth*, a newspaper often reflecting the famous antislavery views of William Lloyd Garrison's newspaper, and choosing for her book publisher the vehement James Redpath, "a fiery abolitionist" (Stern, Introduction, *Letters* xxv).

26. Even in the revised 1869 *Hospital Sketches* Alcott was still concerned with pleasing her readers, explaining in her journal that she was taking out parts that might not win them over: "Anything to suit customers" (*Journals* 164).

27. Elizabeth B. Greene was the illustrator for Alcott's 1868 *Morning-Glories and Other Stories* and may have been tapped by Alcott for the 1869 *Hospital Sketches, and Camp and Fireside Stories*. There are similarities in the illustrations for both books. Even more similar, though, is the work of a Mrs. Innis, at least according to a description of her work by Alcott in a letter to Mary Mapes Dodge (about 1874; Stern is unsure of the date): "I like Mrs Innis' drawing better than Miss Greene's. Mrs. I is illustrating a book for me now. . . . Her children are altogether charm-

ing, thier [*sic*] little fat legs captivate me entirely." Alcott, though, was quick to add, "But I love E. B. G. & don't mind her infant's dropsical heads very much" (Stern, *Louisa May Alcott* 220).

28. I will discuss in Chapter 6 the controversial third principle, first articulated by Frankenberg as "a set of cultural practices that are usually unmarked and unnamed," but which she subsequently changed.

29. Laundering was a job women of all races saw as the most onerous and taxing of the mid-nineteenth century; privileged and middle-class working women systematically turned the backbreaking labor over to women of the working class.

30. Just prior to the New Year's Eve of the Emancipation Proclamation, Alcott had become ill with the beginnings of what proved to be an almost fatal case of typhoid fever. When she jumped out of bed and electrified her roommate, she probably surprised her in part because Alcott had been ordered to strict bed rest.

31. Frederick Douglass also described a scene of celebration, stating, "I never saw Joy before," as men and women of all ages threw hats up in the air (Douglass, *Life and Writings* 337).

Chapter Two

1. Georgeanna Woolsey served in other locations besides Gettysburg, for instance at the emergency hospital set up at the Patent Office in Washington, DC, and on the hospital ship USS *Daniel Webster* in 1862. She went on to marry Dr. Frank Bacon in 1866, whom she knew from before the war.

2. Woolsey and her mother had gone to Gettysburg "under the impression, due to a mistake in telegraphing, that Charley [Georgeanna's brother] was hurt; and, being on hand, were fastened upon by Mr. [Frederick Law] Olmsted [General Secretary of the United States Sanitary Commission] to take charge of a feeding station and lodge for the wounded men. So there we were, looking after other people's boys, since our own was safe" (Woolsey, Hoisington 312).

3. For instance, see my "Civil War Nursing Narratives" in the *Walt Whitman Quarterly Review*.

Chapter Three

1. C. appeared several times in *Notes of Hospital Life*, especially near the beginnings of chapters, primarily to serve as a reminder of the "woman question" and to function as proxy for the reader. On at least one occasion, though, the character of C. did not function this way, given the familiar and slightly suspenseful tone Dunlap adopted when she addressed her, saying that she hoped C. had

enjoyed the sunshiny day, but as for herself, she had done something different: "I escaped from my duties here for one hour and spent it you know where" (43). C. apparently knew how Dunlap had spent her unaccounted-for hour, but the cagey Dunlap withheld that information from readers. Given that she mentioned the visit of the Bishop of Minnesota directly afterward in the same paragraph, it may have been an in-joke between the two women about congregational matters.

2. That Dunlap would use fictional devices such as this comes as no surprise, given that soon after the war she published a piece of fiction in *Godey's Lady's Book*, in 1867. The story carried the name of Julia Dunlap, and was entitled "Aunt Patty; Or, the Endowment." This story tackled Dunlap's prevailing subject of wealth and the lack of it, with the characters of a rich aunt and a middle-class young woman affianced to a man who needed money to get married. It also carried clear hallmarks in the hostess-like narrator directing the reader to "listen to the conversation in that corner" (320), as well as presenting a narrator interested in "powers of observation"(322). The same fictional device of hostess narrator is also prominent in the 1870 children's book, *Under the Holly*, co-written with Margaret Hosmer and published by a Philadelphia press.

3. In this offering, for instance, Dunlap intoned about the "Chastening Hand" and the "Sword of Prayer," among many other sermonic elements (see pp. 123–127).

4. She may have counseled Temperance, especially as that was one of Bishop Potter's primary causes.

5. It is possible she told on herself because she thought it might be instructive to her readers' own attempts at converting others.

6. Later, however, after Darlington eventually passed away, Dunlap presented Christian words of comfort to the reader. Interestingly, Dunlap concluded the tale by mentioning a male nurse named Richards, who had a "kinder heart," she said, than anyone. Though he was considered an indifferent nurse when he lacked a connection with the patient, he was one of the best when "he had a special interest," as he did "in the highest degree" with Darlington (88). Dunlap spoke at some length about the relationship between the two men, saying she had often "wondered at the tender love which seemed to exist between them" (88). She tried to give solace to Richards, who needed it in mourning Darlington's passing, and when she comforted him, she did not borrow from religious adages. She admired the male nurse's ability to form genuine connections with his patients.

7. She ended the chapter with a poem, probably of her own composition, containing many particulars from the chapter, such as her laying on of hands: "Cooled was his burning brain/By loving hands" (91). Though it used words of Christian sentiment, it also showed remarkably personal details.

8. In another incident with the patient Gavin, Dunlap broke from Christian rhetoric to insert a story rich in the elements of romantic fiction. Dunlap discovered, to her consternation, while running an errand, that Gavin was languishing in a stairwell, as she "stumble[d] upon something on the stair" (106). This contrasted with his appearance when she first saw him and he displayed an "erect and military bearing, well-made figure, and broad chest, with the certain 'je ne sais quoi' of a gentleman" (106). Dunlap was taken with Gavin's "interesting melancholy" and "large, dark eyes" (107) to the point that her friend M. had teased her about him: "'Oh! You want to make up a romantic story for him, do you?'" (107). Dunlap's encounter with Gavin had the added intrigue that he came from a split North–South heritage. The scene of tripping over him on the steps was imbued with a forbidden quality, set as it was in a dim, liminal space apart from the accepted places for interaction between nurse and patient. He also confided in Dunlap an as-yet untold secret. The eroticized Gavin brought out Dunlap's affinity for the pulp novel, and when M. teased her a second time about her love of story, Dunlap responded in terms of subliminal passion: "'Story! He never opens his lips to any one; and unless he shall need something, I have almost determined never to open mine to him again'" (109). Dunlap convinced Gavin that unloading his heart to her about his melancholy was as important as unbuckling his knapsack from his injured back. The tale held the most intensive display of desire in the memoir. Dunlap refrained from packaging the lesson in Christian discourse.

9. Nightingale suggested that the tool most successful in nursing was the act of observation, a multifaceted cognitive act, whereby a nurse would daily survey her patients: "what to observe—how to observe—what symptoms indicate improvement—what the reverse—which are of importance—which are of none—which are the evidence of neglect—and of what kind of neglect" (105). Nightingale contrasted these layered powers of feminine observation with the kind of observation, for example, proffered in a court of law. In court, anyone can be believed to speak the whole truth, but "it requires many faculties combined of observation and memory to speak 'the whole truth,' and to say 'nothing but the truth'" (106), an ability she marked as female. Her refined sense of gendered perception allowed women nurses to make a singular contribution to the history of medicine. Observation as a womanly mainstay occupied the energies of all nurses studied here, as they applied close observation to the their labor, as well as to their compositional practice.

10. Dunlap knew the proclivities of her particular friend, C., and when she later she asked C. if she would like to take that "long-promised trip through the wards," she guaranteed that her friend would be shielded from any of the "'horrors of hospital life. You shall not see an open wound if I can help it'" (168).

Robert Leigh Davis mentions that, "many Civil War nursing narratives disclaim direct representations of suffering . . . [as] an anonymous nurse writes in *Notes of Hospital Life* . . ." (109). Davis's observation applies to Dunlap, but not to some others that describe suffering explicitly.

11. Further, Dunlap claimed the woman used the visit as an opportunity to try to "extort funds" from Dunlap (135).

12. Dunlap showed her tolerance in a slightly different way in the account she gave of the presence of a rebel in the hospital, and of the group of local women who arrived to gawk at him. This scene, anticipated by Georgeanna Woolsey's tale of the Dutch man who wanted to see rebels at Gettysburg, saw Dunlap championing the equality of people from different regions. In protecting a Confederate soldier, Dunlap defended the everyman: "I can assure you that he is exactly like any of these men you see around you; were you to go into the ward you could not distinguish him, unless he were pointed out to you" (34). She denied the women access to the man, seeing their motivations as "morbid curiosity" (36).

13. It is important to note the caveat, though, that this conventional disclaimer for women authors—that they shirked none of their feminine duties in writing a book—had been used in regard to American female authors for centuries, from Anne Bradstreet to Mary Rowlandson to Phyllis Wheatley.

14. The Episcopal Church stated its objective as one in which the church members joined in gratitude "to God for rearing up an Institution which cares for the soul's eternal interests, whilst the body is being restored to health. All the inmates of the Hospital have been reached and benefitted by this pervading religious influence, and many of them have openly confessed Christ in baptism or confirmation" (*Woman's* 15).

15. Schultz, however, posits another reason that some nurses chose authorial obscurity: "Scores of women helped support themselves by publishing accounts of wartime work, but few would have admitted they were writing for living expenses" (162).

Chapter Four

1. Powers was also modest in claiming the value of the daily "minutia [*sic*] of hospital service" (v) as an alternative to the heroic memoir, stating simplicity and immediacy as her aesthetic principles, writing about only what occurred as she observed it. In the usual convention of referring to women writers, though, she added that she would "neglect no duty for the sake of scribbling about it" (2).

2. She was from North Oxford, Massachusetts (Schultz 236).

3. Powers made notations, for instance, on the linden, ailanthus, daffodil (5),

hyacinth, crocus, peach (13), pomegranate flower (23), apple, japonica (59), tulip tree, and sycamore (98).

4. He may have gleaned the gist of this joke from a cartoon, "Rubbing It In—Scene in the Park Barracks" from an 1862 edition of *Frank Leslie's Illustrated Newspaper*.

5. With this portrait, Powers anticipated a later narrative segment in which she gave approval and admiration to the "15th Colored Regiment performing peerlessly at dress parade" (79).

6. Drawing on the history of civil disobedience as a basis for abolition, Powers recalled especially the Massachusetts resident Thoreau, with whose concepts she might well have been familiar.

7. Pivotal to liberal Northerners was the response of Bostonians and other Massachusetts residents to the reviled 1850 Fugitive Slave Law, which in effect made criminals of those who aided or harbored escaping slaves.

8. The man was "Hickman Nutter, of the 31st Ohio" (19).

9. In the chapter on Sophronia Bucklin's *In Hospital and Camp*, we see Bucklin engaging in four basic tactics of dissent: interpretation, appeal, noncompliance, and confrontation.

10. Not only did Powers work in the smallpox ward; she worked in the gangrene tent in Indiana, where she visited four of her patients who had been transferred there. Explaining to the reader that they had been given an "impure vaccination, and now the gangrene has appeared," she added, "it is said to be worse than a wound to heal" (121). The patients with the three worst cases complained that the smell of their wounds nauseated them constantly, so she made handkerchiefs to douse with cologne. Before visiting the tents she "never saw or scarcely imagined such suffering" (123), especially when bromine was applied to the wounds. Powers attempted to help during one such treatment by holding a man's swollen elbow in her hand while "the nurse proceeded to take off the oakum which had been saturated with bromine, and then to pick off from the side of the raw wound, the burnt pieces of flesh, with a pair of pincers," upon which the man began "to cry for mercy" (124). Almost fainting, Powers dropped the man's arm into the hand of another nurse, and everyone—even the patient—laughed good-naturedly at her.

11. To accomplish many of her feats Bickerdyke used the figure of the mother as moral authority for her actions, as did nurses in general, but Bickerdyke was the most famous and prominent American exemplar of that authority. She once attempted to track a shipment of fruits and vegetables for her soldiers and found it sidetracked on the rails: "'those cars of vegetables moved on to a side track to *spoil for days*, while some of these officers have been sending on their *fine furniture to keep house with* . . . '" Bickerdyke told the "'fine gentleman in shoulder-straps"

to put the vegetables back on track and "send on those things in double quick-time, or I'd have his official head taken off. And I asked him if it needed a Miss Nancy to come and tell Miss Betty what her duty was, before she could do it'" (75). Powers admired Bickerdyke's bombast, but retained her own slightly caustic, ironic tone, for example, when she commented on General Sherman's pronouncement on women. Sherman had denigrated women nurses when one of his officers queried him as to whether he would allow a woman nurse to accompany the troops, saying, "'Send always a barrel of pork, in place of a woman!'" (103). Powers's dry riposte was, "The General is intensely complimentary" (103).

12. Powers also had high commendations for her friend Annie Bell, mentioned above. Bell, a matron at the Nashville Hospital, was "an amiable, self-reliant, educated lady & consciencious [*sic*] Christian" (Moore, *Papers* 5); Bell was also "a self--reliant, judicious, pure & noble woman & indefatigable worker for our Union invalid soldiers" (6).

13. Another incident did not involve bureaucratic red tape but showed similar gender scapegoating; Powers was falsely accused by a patient who thought she had reported him for drunkenness. She wrote back to him that he had mistakenly assumed she reported him, suggesting that he wrongly presupposed gender when he implied, "'the *woman* that was given to be with us, *she* did it?'" (125). In other words, the man attempted to blame Powers for his own drunkenness, passing off to her the responsibility for his infraction. His actions evidenced an outgrowth of a system that had internalized prejudice against women.

14. She showed stiff resistance to authorities' misuse of power, indignant at "multiform abuses" (210), one of which included the deplorable mistakes she found in reports, such as the man "who was detailed for light duty" though he was in the dead house (168). Another was the fact that she was reprimanded for accompanying a corporal fifteen years her junior to church, an act for which she "came very near being discharged" (157–8). She was especially rankled by the misuse of donations and funds designated for books for patients, her pet cause; Powers felt outrage because several hundred books expressly for patients were kept boxed up until the end of the war even though "several thousands of dollars" had been given also for the enterprise of organizing a reading room (203).

15. In addition, Powers, staying in a Nashville residence, spoke with the former housekeeper, Aunt Nanny, who told her an anecdote exemplifying the black community's organization, efficacy, and camaraderie as they kept confidence among themselves to deceive the city's white population. When the Union forces entered Nashville, the white people heard the news of the coming invasion Sunday morning on their way to church, but as Aunt Nanny related, the enslaved people, through their own channels of communication, already "'knew it in the night'" (70).

16. Powers recorded yet another story of a woman, Aunt Nancy, who predated the character of Aunt Rachel in Mark Twain's heralded "A True Story." In Twain's tale, Aunt Rachel, a former slave, responded to the white narrator's comment that she had never had any trouble, and she set him straight that she had had both great trouble and great joy. In Powers's telling of Aunt Nancy's story, the former bondswoman, similarly told by a white person that she'd never had any trouble, replied, "'may be I don' know what trouble is, but my old man was sold away from me down in old Virginny . . . and then my son . . . my last little boy an' girl . . . an' now I'm getting so old I'll never go back to ole Virginny any more!'" (69). Twain claimed that his "A True Story" was set down more or less just as it transpired; Powers's story, predating his, shows that variations on the tale had been in circulation for some time.

Chapter Five

1. Holstein returned to Merion after the war, and in 1892 received a pension of $12 a month; she died in 1900 (Conklin 264).

2. Bespeaking urgency, her paragraphs eschewed transition as episodes plunged from one to the next, sentences at times standing as predicative constructions lacking a subject.

3. She offered an acerbic description of a former slaveholder who complained he no longer had any enslaved people to work his crops and lamented that his crop of corn could not be harvested. Holstein, hearing later that the Union cavalry had foraged in the man's cornfield, observed summarily to her reader that the slaveholder "was spared further trouble [of worrying about the harvest] on that score" (64).

4. In Holstein's narrative several black laborers worked at jobs different from those usually described by other nurse narrators, as in the case of the black man entrusted with the important job of gridding a cemetery to protect the names of the interred against loss of identity (in case Confederate soldiers destroyed markers). Elsewhere she stated that freedmen manned a steam fire-engine used to keep down the camp dust and cool the tents: "a large force of negroes have it in charge, and already the good results are seen" (80).

5. As did Woolsey and others, Holstein portrayed "contrabands" in clichéd ways, such in the stereotype of them singing and praying "in the most devout manner" (81).

6. In addition, the paragraph ended with a gendered concession to female bravery, including Southern females, for among the prisoners "is a rebel woman, sergeant of artillery—she was the last to leave the gun when captured" (72). The paragraph contained many evolving cultural perceptions of race and gender.

7. The ensuing remove was a grueling passage (with several soldiers running by the side of an ambulance to keep it steady), of several days' length, during which they passed more scenes of destruction. One bizarre incident, however, turned out to be a kind of recycling rather than a waste: the troops came upon cavalry horses left behind by Northern troops a couple of days ahead of Holstein's group. Her group reclaimed them, as the animals had had time to rest. They controlled the horses with bridles made of tent canvas and saddles made of blankets.

8. Holstein detailed, accurately, that most of the lives lost in the explosion were those of "colored laborers" (86).

9. Distinct from the experience of, say, Alcott, whose duties were confined to the daily schedules of one hospital in one city—or at least gave the illusion of structure, until the wounded arrived—Holstein's regimen was so unregulated that, because of her "hurried, continued work," she claimed it was "impossible to give an exact account of even one day's labor" (68). By referring to "one day's labor," Holstein may have contrasted her experience with the *Hospital Sketches*' chapter, "One Day," in which Alcott showed the activities undertaken by the woman nurse in a twenty-four-hour period.

10. Elsewhere, Bucklin found she had trouble crossing from military to civilian life. At one point, soon after having taken part in a military funeral ceremony, Holstein returned to society for a wedding ceremony, and afterwards could only think how the food at that event could have been used more efficiently at the front (18).

11. Other women nurses left a record of their opinion of Holstein's work at Gettysburg, especially concerning her position of some power. Weighing in on her administrative style, Cornelia Hancock wrote that, "I like Mrs. Holstein real well. I am most too smart for her. I *will* get the things for the men without orders and she is a great respecter of order" (23). Bucklin also made a somewhat similar observation, though without the sanguine qualifiers, seeing "Mrs. Holstein" as too great a stickler for order, to the point of withholding food from the men by keeping the kitchen off limits to others, as when Holstein placed a "guard, with fixed bayonet, at the entrance" (175). As counterweight to the above, Fisher and Rex (who were not at Gettysburg), in their essay on Pennsylvania women observed that "Mrs. Holstein's lovely, serene countenance indicated power as well as piety" (166).

12. Faust writes extensively about Civil War watchfulness concerning death rituals and the material importance of the body, even after burial: "Redemption and resurrection of the body were understood as physical, not just metaphysical, realities, and therefore the body, even in death and dissolution, preserved 'a surviving identity'" (62).

13. In fact, Holstein's conjoining of military and domestic images conflated

the strange and familiar in a combination that recalled the condition for gothic literature—Freud's uncanny, or *Unheimliche*, the circumstances under which experience that most haunts a subject is that which is most familiar. As the warfront and homefront converged, those things closest to home could become those that were most "unhomely," or strange. Obviously, Holstein was not a gothic writer, but she used a tone difficult to pin down, the uncanny elements of her voice representing experience that resisted representation.

14. In another such tale, a young lieutenant had passed away quietly in the hospital, until a glee club entered, singing "Rally Round the Flag," at which point, the lieutenant, alive after all, "sprang up, exclaiming, 'Yes, boys, we did 'rally round the flag,'" before he passed away for the "final" time (48).

15. Such lingering on suffering is what some contemporary commentators might call "misery porn," which presents a legitimate problem for any writer discoursing on events that are agonizing to articulate and socially unacceptable to detail at extreme length.

16. As an aside, Holstein reported that the medical community was baffled as to how to treat the starvation of the prisoners of war because extreme privation was so rare in civilian life that medical books did not include it.

17. Holstein, however, lived a long and fruitful life in the decades after the war, active in civic duties as an organizer in the Daughters of the American Revolution, working on purchasing and commemorating Valley Forge (*Daughters of the American Revolution Magazine* 179).

Chapter Six

1. Leonard states that Bucklin, an unmarried seamstress, "belonged neither to the elite nor to the working class" (5).

2. It is possible, too, that Bucklin wrote the original with an extra word, "men," and later crossed it out, but even so, the slip showed that the word "selfish" occurred as a considered decision she wanted to keep.

3. Leonard also postulates that Bucklin's narrative was gender-driven, though not expressly in relation to the "Declaration."

4. Bucklin was not alone, of course, in perceiving graft. David Williams records that "a single congressional committee discovered up to $50 million in losses to the public treasury from government contract frauds" (104).

5. As one political theorist asserts, "the central question in any discussion of civil disobedience concerns the point at which it becomes morally permissible—or even obligatory—to resist the authority of unjust laws or institutions" (Tebbit 102).

6. Bucklin mentioned other infractions, among them extortion, unorthodox

punishments, profiteering, drunkenness on duty, and potential medical abuses, such as possibly unnecessary amputation. About one amputation Bucklin reported: "I shall never outlive the feeling that [the soldier's] was an unnecessary amputation . . . his wound was only that of a bullet through the fleshy part of the arm. After the amputation, which did not discharge properly, his symptoms grew fatal, and when he died, seven or eight days afterwards, he was bloated to a misshapen, monstrous size, whilst his body was almost as transparent as glass" (108–09). About drunkenness, Bucklin reported: "There were men, in whose presence you felt as if a whisky barrel was well represented, who had to be approached with all the deference due the insignia of office represented by their shoulder-straps. Often we felt that it was an insult to our womanhood to be constrained to give an outward show of respect when within there was nothing but loathing and detestation" (175–76). One such surgeon arrived in the ward at night, staggering to the point that he needed to hold the tent-pole, and cursed the workers, "declaring he could not understand why the nurses had not uncovered the wounds for him to examine" (176).

7. In this debriefing with the superintendent, Bucklin remembered that Dix had previously cautioned her, possibly with innuendo, about a strange situation existing also at Camp Stoneman; additionally, Bucklin remembered another case in which there was a "suspicious woman, who had no duties to perform in the hospital" (241).

8. It is worth noting that Bucklin was punished for her disobedience in many ways, but one of the more surreptitious of punishments included compelling her to sew—a job she detested: "stitching aimlessly at tattered garments was not my work. The flush of indignation mantled my cheek, when I thought of the treatment to which loyal women had been subjected . . ." (128). Reprimanded for infractions against the military hierarchy and compelled to work at sewing, Bucklin may at times have been the recipient of a message implying that she should stay within the realm of harmless "women's" work.

9. Bucklin took pains to distance herself from the sanctimonious posturing and power abuse of the top brass, even mocking officers' attempts to reinforce authority through their costume, as they "draw up the white paper collars which surmounted their bright uniforms, as though conscious of inspiring respect by the show of seeming linen" (70). (Indeed, Bucklin was very aware of the potential haughtiness of both genders, given that she scorned the pretentions of upper-class women as well, as when they attempted to perform the labor of nursing with "gloves on jewelled hands" [125].)

10. As a gauge of the role of gender in the wages for nurses, consider that at the beginning of the Civil War women nurses were paid $12 per month, compared with the $20.50 paid to "their male counterparts" (Oates 22).

11. Money, a constant topic, was also broached when Chase mentioned an indigent friend or family member who didn't write, she suspected, "because they cant [*sic*] spare the three cents."

12. I mark here the coincidence that the letters of the moniker S. L. C. coincide with the letters of the name of Sylvia Lawson Covey, who wrote the preface to the text of Sarah A. Palmer, *The Story of Aunt Becky's Army-life*, and that both writers used powerful rhetoric to defend the working-class nurse, wielding the most fiery diction contained in the twelve nurse narratives of this period. (Both Bucklin and Palmer were from proximate counties in New York, Bucklin from Auburn in Cayuga County, and Palmer from Ithaca in Tompkins County.) Stylistically they were similar, too: S. L. C. ended her introduction to Bucklin's narrative by making a gesture of handing the book over to an audience she encouraged to be "discriminating," and Sylvia Lawson Covey ended her preface to Palmer's book by handing it over with an announcer's flair, exhorting the audience in her final words to be "a generous public, which will not fail to deal fairly, the pages of this unpretending Story of Aunt Becky's Army Life" (vii); both finished with the title of the book in the crescendo of the final sentence. Both S. L. C. and Sylvia Lawson Covey stated that the respective nurse they were introducing received from the common soldier "scores of letters" and "numerous" testimonials (Bucklin 27 / Palmer iv); both favored several words, as for instance "bejeweled" hands / "jeweled hand" (Bucklin 29 / Palmer v), and "unpretending" (Bucklin 30 / Palmer iii). Sizer notes that the two may be the same (304), and I concur. Covey was a published sonneteer.

13. Frankenberg's revision of the third principle takes into account the important circumstance that "the notion of whiteness as unmarked norm is revealed to be a mirage or indeed, to put it even more strongly, a white delusion" (*The Mirage of an Unmarked Whiteness* 73), which is to say that the inimical whiteness, with the white presumption of advantage, is in fact highly visible, especially to those not wielding the advantage.

14. Judging the women's attitude about the ruined bedding to be careless, Bucklin neglected the probability that they had not been told of the operation's goals or the extent of the hospital's resources. She had the acuity, though, to comprehend that from their perspective the hospital resources might have seemed "inexhaustible" compared with their previous lack of resources when enslaved.

15 Interestingly, this matron against whom Bucklin fumed was presented very differently by the Woolseys; see Hoisington 321, 344, 350.

16. Bucklin may invoke the term greybacks, "a humorous name for lice" (Wright, *Language* 133), to indicate class parity, given that everyone is infested alike.

17. Another point of mutuality between races occurred afterward, when Bucklin attended a reunion with some of the black troops.

Chapter Seven

1. Georgeanna Woolsey's experience was similar to the extent that she went looking for her brother whom she also thought was wounded, but unlike Wheelock, found him in good health and stayed on (see Chapter 2).

2. The local papers kept up with Wheelock after the war, too, albeit in a small way: the *Jackson Citizen Patriot* announced that bills in the Senate and House were "providing a pension for Julia Wheelock Freeman" (Jan 21, 1889, 7). The *Bay City Times* likewise reported the pension awarded the "noted Michigan nurse, at $25 a month" (Jan 26, 1889, 2).

3. In fact, Wheelock mentioned helping soldiers from many states, including Massachusetts, New York, and Pennsylvania, among others. She also wrote that without the succor of New York, Maryland, Pennsylvania, and Maine relief organizations, the Michigan operation "would almost entirely have ceased" (136).

4. Interestingly, Wheelock's diary made mention of the "three sick men" (1:22; Dec 18, 1862), but not of her activism and dissent in taking the initiative in speaking to Dr. Curtis. Her diary does, however, mention an even more assertive and potentially dissenting opinion, in which she used very strong diction to report news that made her question her government. She related that she had received "a letter from Reuben Smith conveying the most distressing intelligence—if it should prove true—viz. that brother Homer & his brother Ansel & many others of their Reg were to be hung, for refusing to work any longer without pay—they have been in the service about 15 months & have not been paid anything yet,—but can it be that our Government will permit 200 or more of its brave boys to be hung on such grounds as that; if so my confidence in our government is for one shaken" (1:23; Dec 18, 1862). Distressed in her diary, she nonetheless chose not to follow this tack in the book.

5. She helped other men to leave Camp Convalescent in addition to those discussed above, either by seeing that they were "admitted to the 'Examining Board' for discharge" or admitted to the Fairfax Street Hospital.

6. None of this is to suggest that Wheelock was a lone crusader in the matter of Camp Convalescent; in fact, another nurse, Amy Morris Bradley, from Maine, was "the prime mover in reforming Alexandria's convalescent camp, where she spoke for five thousand soldiers" (Schultz 2).

7. Wheelock mentioned the incident, too, in her diary, and went further than in the book by naming the surgeon, Dr. Boice: "Had a talk with Dr. Boice in regard to the rude manner in which he treated me a few days before . . ." (1:19–20:

Dec 6, 1862). On the other hand, the book went further than the diary in drawing conclusions about the doctor's behavior toward female workers.

8. Other narratives were based on diaries, too, as for instance, Powers's narrative, which she undoubtedly transformed for public consumption, given the polish of her work.

9. Wheelock was a well-educated young woman whose attendance at Kalamazoo College would have prepared her to record her observations. In the Kalamazoo College Catalogue for the years 1858–1859, she was listed as being from Wesleyville, Pennsylvania, and in the "second collegiate year" (Catalogue 16). There were sixteen women in her class, mostly from Michigan, especially southwest Michigan around Kalamazoo, but also from the states of Illinois, Vermont, and of course Pennsylvania. Her education consisted of extensive reading in Latin, French, and English, as well as additional studies in subjects such as "Book Keeping, Plane Geometry, Biblical History, Composition, Drawing, and Vocal Music" (Catalogue 25). The rationale for study at the college was plainly stated: "The object aimed at is the development of true and noble womanhood" (Catalogue 29).

10. Wheelock's strikethroughs and underlinings are purposely shown here.

11. Wheelock still felt the need to protect the reputation of the female nurse in the 1870 *The Boys in White*, even though it was published five years after the end of the Civil War.

12. She copied the verse on the back of manuscript page 26 instead of page 25 probably because the paper was in coupled sheets. Wheelock added other verses as well, as for instance on manuscript page 29, with a first attempt at the addition on the back of page 29, subsequently crossed out, the final candidate for addition on the back of page 30.

13. Wheelock did, however rarely, paste an entry sideways, as on page 81 of the scrapbook, where she presented a poem, James Russell Lowell's "Concord Ode" in its entirety, except for the final lines, which she finished by placing vertically in the right margin.

14. Only three of the pages in the scrapbook are blank.

15. A preponderance of the stanzas have to do with consolation and related themes such as fallen heroes, orphans, the mourning of soldiers, mother, home, and patriotism. The clippings, not presented chronologically, were gleaned largely from publications of the 1860s, with some from the late 1850s and some from the early 1870s. At times Wheelock seemed to identify a theme for a couple of pages; for instance, one page contains mostly clippings about Lincoln (Scrapbook 9), while another is covered with prose clippings (45), and another one-and-a-half pages are reserved exclusively for Adoniram Judson (pages 84–85), a Baptist missionary. The last four pages of the scrapbook are devoted to re-

views of *The Boys in White*. Even the occasional theme page most often thins out thematically at the bottom of the page, where considerations of space seem to trump content. The material at the bottom is characterized by small rectangles of clippings, containing maxims and epigrams concerning, say, promises, the trials of life, or politeness.

16. It is possible, also, that the words written on the poems may have been added by someone other than Wheelock before the poems were given to her, or when she shared the scrapbook with a friend.

17. Handwritten on top of the reward, curiously, is a note: "Please accept this as a New Years [*sic*] present it is all I have with me at present to give EBR" (113).

18. She cut verse from magazines as varied as *The Atlantic Monthly*, *Moore's Rural New Yorker*, *The New York Tribune*, and *The Christian Herald*, representing poets such as John Greenleaf Whittier, Elizabeth Barrett Browning, William Cullen Bryant, and Ella Wheeler Wilcox.

19. Wheelock wished her narrative might be metaphorically "embalmed," but she referred to embalming for another, much more literal reason. Civil War funeral practices were a matter of great concern to mid-century Americans, and embalming was a relatively novel and expensive operation compared to conventional burial, but families occasionally chose it as the means to transport the bodies of their loved ones home. (The procedure was used even more after Abraham Lincoln's 1865 embalmment, by which "the president's paraded body was deified, a source of healing for the wounded nation" (Grimes 265). Wheelock may have mentioned embalming as a way to suggest national healing, but given that families of the common soldier (such as her family) could probably not afford the procedure, she bespoke, possibly, an inability to preserve the body of her brother and, obliquely, an inability to honor him fully.

20. Wheelock's narrative exhibited some tonal similarities to Phelps's *The Gates Ajar*, wherein the speaker received a letter about her brother in the army, tried to face his loss, doubted the comforts of faith, looked askance at "that most exquisite of inquisitions, the condolence system" (5), and could not shake "the bare, blank sense of physical repulsion from death" (7).

21. She used this phrase in recounting the experience of a dying patient.

22. One of Wheelock's strikingly memorable observations of Lincoln's funeral procession was that "the trees were filled with weeping spectators" (256).

23. For eight years after the war, Wheelock worked in Washington at the Treasury Department, then returned to Michigan in 1873 and married Porter C. Freeman, giving birth to two sons in 1876 and 1879 (Pferdehirt 44).

24. One of these four sentences is spectacularly conciliatory, justifying the war as follows: "the three hundred thousand graves where sleep the 'Boys in White' were not made in vain'" (267). However, if we had to weigh the 300,000

graves as justification against the repeated phrase "boys in white," with its accumulating overtones of futility, it might prove painful.

Conclusion

1. In general, national conflicts accelerate labor gains but are not lasting, as Baxandall, Gordon, and Reverby assert: "The increase in women's employment and the debate this engenders is always exacerbated by wars. The extraordinary labors of women in the Civil War were for the most part temporary . . ." (75).

2. Albeit writing about English authors, Catherine Judd asserts similarly that the nineteenth-century female nurse was a figure who "develops as a category for perceptions about gender and class, consolidating for the Victorian writer fundamental political and social anxieties—especially concerns over class conflict, public health, the Woman Question, female heroics, and the construction of middle-class sexuality" (2).

3. On the last page of her book about suffering, Faust asserts, "We still live in the world of death the Civil War created" (271), meaning that although we have progressed to become more attentive to formal burials for the dead, and although we have curtailed the nineteenth-century failures to identify the dead, the larger picture remains; namely, the Civil War subsumed the soldier into a great bureaucracy and inhumanity, and contemporary warfare has only escalated that level of bureaucracy and sense of meaninglessness. The nurse memoirist animated the concerns of preserving humanity and self as she witnessed in person the great number of lives shattered and lost.

4. As Litosseliti and Sunderland attest, the study of discourse and the study of gender are yoked, in that "a discourse approach to gender and language aims to accommodate ideas of individual agency, and of gender (identity) as multiple, fluctuating, and shaped in part by language" (6).

BIBLIOGRAPHY

Adams, John Greenleaf. *Fifty Notable Years: Views of the Ministry of Christian Universalism.* Boston: Universalist Publishing House, 1882.

Alcott, Louisa May. *Hospital Sketches.* Ed. Elaine Showalter. *Alternative Alcott.* New Brunswick: Rutgers University Press, 1988. 3–73.

———. "Hospital Sketches, I–IV." *The Commonwealth.* May 22, 1863; May 29, 1863; June 12, 1863; June 26, 1863.

———. *Hospital Sketches, and Camp and Fireside Stories.* Boston: Roberts Brothers, 1869.

———. *The Journals of Louisa May Alcott.* Eds. Joel Myerson, Daniel Shealy, and Madeleine B. Stern. Boston: Little, Brown, 1989.

———. *Louisa May Alcott: Her Life, Letters, and Journals.* Ed. Edna D. Cheney. Boston: Little, Brown, 1919.

———. *The Selected Letters of Louisa May Alcott.* Eds. Joel Myerson, Daniel Shealy, and Madeleine B. Stern. Boston: Little, Brown, 1987.

Alkana, Joseph. "Introduction: Cohesion, Dissent, and the Aims of Criticism." Eds. Carol Colatrella and Joseph Alkana. *Cohesion and Dissent In America.* Albany: State University of New York Press, 1994. ix–xxi.

American Literary Gazette and Publishers' Circular. Advertisement. Sept 1, 1863. 1, 9, 346.

Ammons, Elizabeth. Foreword. *White Women in Racialized Spaces: Imaginative Transformation and Ethical Action in Literature.* Eds. Samina Najmi and Rajini Srikanth. Albany: State University of New York Press, 2002. ix–x.

Arac, Jonathan. *The Emergence of American Literary Narrative, 1820–1860.* Cambridge, MA: Harvard University Press, 2005.

Attie, Jeanie. *Patriotic Toil: Northern Women and the American Civil War.* Ithaca, NY: Cornell University Press, 1998.

Austin, Anne L. *The Woolsey Sisters of New York: A Family's Involvement in the Civil War and a New Profession (1860–1900).* Philadelphia: American Philosophical Society, 1971.

Austin, John Longshaw. *How to Do Things with Words.* Cambridge, MA: Harvard University Press, 1975.

Bacon, Georgeanna Woolsey and Eliza Woolsey Howland. *My Heart Toward Home: Letters of a Family During the Civil War*. Ed. Daniel John Hoisington. Roseville, MN: Edinborough Press, 2001.

Bacon, Jacqueline. *The Humblest May Stand Forth: Rhetoric, Empowerment, and Abolition*. Columbia: University of South Carolina Press, 2002.

Barrett Browning, Elizabeth. *Aurora Leigh and Other Poems*. Eds. John Robert Glorney Bolton and Julia Bolton Holloway. New York: Penguin, 1995.

Baxandall, Rosalyn Fraad, Linda Gordon, and Susan Reverby. *America's Working Women: A Documentary History, 1600 to the Present*. New York: W. W. Norton, 1995.

Bay City Times (Jan 26, 1889). 7.

Beecher, Catharine. *A Treatise on Domestic Economy, for the Use of Young Ladies at Home, and School*. Boston: Thomas H. Webb, 1843.

Bennett, Paula Bernat. "Subtle Subversion: Mary Louise Booth and *Harper's Bazaar* (1867–1889)." *Blue Pencils and Hidden Hands: Women Editing Periodicals, (1830–1910)*. Eds. Sharon M. Harris and Ellen Gruber Garvey. Boston: Northeastern University Press, 2004. 225–47.

Beschloss, Michael, Ed. *100 Milestone Documents from the National Archives*. New York: Oxford University Press, 2003.

Bercovitch, Sacvan. *The Puritan Origins of the American Self*. New Haven, CT: Yale University Press, 1975.

Berger, Bruce K., and Bryan H. Reber. *Gaining Influence in Public Relations: The Role of Resistance in Practice*. Mahwah, NJ: Lawrence Erlbaum Associates, 2006.

Bhabha, Homi. "The White Stuff." *Artforum*. May 1998, 21–24.

———. *Nation and Narration*. New York: Psychology Press, 1990.

Bleiker, Roland. *Popular Dissent, Human Agency and Global Politics*. Cambridge: Cambridge University Press, 2000.

Blight, David W. *Race and Reunion: The Civil War in American Memory*. Cambridge, MA: Belknap Press, 2001.

Book News: A Monthly Survey of General Literature. Vol. 12. (Sept 1893–Aug 1894). Philadelphia: John Wanamaker, 1894.

Bostridge, Mark. *Florence Nightingale: The Making of an Icon*. New York: Farrar, Straus and Giroux, 2008.

Boudreau, Kristin. *Sympathy in American Literature: American Sentiments from Jefferson to the Jameses*. Gainesville: University Press of Florida, 2002.

Breitweiser, Mitchell Robert. *American Puritanism and the Defense of Mourning: Religion, Grief, and Ethnology in Mary White Rowlandson's Captivity Narrative*. Madison: University of Wisconsin Press, 1990.

Brekus, Catherine. *Strangers and Pilgrims: Female Preaching in America, 1740–1845*. Chapel Hill: University of North Carolina Press, 1998.

Brockett, Linus Pierpont. *The Camp, the Battlefield, and the Hospital; Or, Lights and Shadows of the Great Rebellion*. Philadelphia: National Publishing Company, 1866.

Brockett, L. P., and Mrs. Mary C. Vaughan. *Woman's Work in the Civil War: A Record of Heroism, Patriotism and Patience*. Philadelphia: Zeigler, McCurdy and Company, 1868.

Brooks, Noah. *Washington in Lincoln's Time*. New York: Century Company, 1895.

Brooks, Stewart. *Civil War Medicine*. Springfield: Charles C. Thomas, 1966.

Brown, Bill. *A Sense of Things: The Object Matter of American Literature*. Chicago: University of Chicago Press, 2003.

Brown, Matthew D. "Reading and National Identity: 1820–1860." *Cultural History of Reading*. Ed. Sarah Quay. Westport: Greenwood Press, 2008.

Brown, Michael Patterson. "Sharing a Sense of Justice: The Role of Conscience in Political Protest." *Spiritual and Political Dimensions of Nonviolence and Peace*. Eds. David Boersema and Katy Gray Brown. New York: Rodopi, 2006. 145–60.

Brown, Thomas J. *Dorothea Dix: New England Reformer*. Cambridge: Harvard University Press, 1998.

Brumgardt, John, Ed. Introduction. *Civil War Nurse: The Diary and Letters of Hannah Ropes*. Knoxville: University of Tennessee Press, 1980.

Bucklin, Sophronia E. *In Hospital and Camp: A Woman's Record of Thrilling Incidents Among the Wounded in the Late War*. Philadelphia: John E. Potter, 1869.

———. Sophronia Bucklin Papers. The History Center in Tompkins County. Ithaca, New York. Folders 1, 7, 8, 21.

Buell, Lawrence. "American Civil War Poetry and the Meaning of Literary Commodification: Whitman, Melville, and Others." *Reciprocal Influences: Literary Production, Distribution, and Consumption in America*. Eds. Steven Fink and Susan S. Williams. Columbus: Ohio State University Press, 1999. 123–38.

Burnham, Michelle. *Captivity and Sentiment: Cultural Exchange in American Literature, 1682–1861*. Hanover: University Press of New England, 1997.

Butler, Judith. *Excitable Speech: A Politics of the Performative*. New York: Psychology Press, 1997.

Carlson, Cheree A. *The Crimes of Womanhood: Defining Femininity in a Court of Law*. Urbana: University of Illinois Press, 2009.

Casper, Scott E. *Constructing American Lives: Biography and Culture in Nineteenth-Century America*. Chapel Hill: University of North Carolina Press, 1999.

Castronovo, Russ. *Necro Citizenship: Death, Eroticism, and the Public Sphere in the Nineteenth-Century United States*. Durham, NC: Duke University Press, 2001.

Catalogue of the Officers and Students of Kalamazoo College, 1858–1859. Kalamazoo: "Telegraph" Book and Job Printing Office, 1859.

Ceniza, Sherry. *Walt Whitman and the Nineteenth-Century Women Reformers*. Tuscaloosa: University of Alabama Press, 1998.

Chambers, John Whiteclay, and Fred Anderson, Eds. *The Oxford Companion to American Military History*. Oxford: Oxford University Press, 1999.

Cheever, Susan. *Louisa May Alcott*. New York: Simon and Schuster, 2010.

Clark, Beverly Lyon. *Louisa May Alcott: The Contemporary Reviews*. West Nyack, NY: Cambridge University Press, 2004.

Claybaugh, Amanda. *The Novel of Purpose: Literature and Social Reform In the Anglo-American World*. Ithaca, NY: Cornell University Press, 2007.

Clinton, Catherine. *The Other Civil War: American Women in the Nineteenth Century*. New York: Hill and Wang, 1999.

———. "'Public Women' and Sexual Politics During the American Civil War." *Battle Scars: Gender and Sexuality In the American Civil War*. Eds. Catherine Clinton and Nina Silber. Oxford: Oxford University Press, 2006. 61–77.

Clinton, Catherine, and Christine Lunardini. *The Columbia Guide to American Women in the Nineteenth Century*. New York: Columbia University Press, 2000.

Conklin, E. F. *Women at Gettysburg 1863*. Gettysburg, PA: Thomas Publications, 1993.

Connecticut Courant. Oct 8, 1864. CI: 5203. 3.

———. June 16, 1866. CII: 5291. 1.

Coogan, Michael David, Marc Zvi Brettler, and Carol A. Newsom, Eds. *The New Annotated Bible, with the Apocrypha*, Augmented 3rd Edition, New Revised Standard Edition. New York: Oxford University Press, 2007.

Creighton, Margaret S. *The Colors of Courage: Gettysburg's Forgotten History: Immigrants, Women, and African Americans in the Civil War's Defining Battle*. New York: Basic Books, 2005.

"Critical Notices." *The North American Review*, Vol. 98. Boston: Crosby and Nichols, 1864. 261–304.

Culpepper, Marilyn Mayer. *All Things Altered: Women in the Wake of Civil War and Reconstruction*. Jefferson, NC: McFarland, 2002.

Cutter, Barbara. *Domestic Devils, Battlefield Angels: The Radicalism of American Womanhood, 1830–1865*. DeKalb: Northern Illinois University Press, 2003.

Daily Eastern Argus. Feb 27, 1865. 33:49. 2.

Dammann, Gordon, and Alfred J. Bollet. *Images of Civil War Medicine: A Photographic History*. New York: Demos Medical Publishing, 2007.

Dannett, Sylvia G. L. *Noble Women of the North*. New York: T. Yoseloff, 1959.

D'Antonio, Patricia. *American Nursing: A History of Knowledge, Authority, and the Meaning of Work*. Baltimore: Johns Hopkins University Press, 2010.
Daughters of the American Revolution Magazine, Vol. 17. National Society of the Daughters of the American Revolution, 1900.
Davis, Cynthia J. *Bodily and Narrative Forms: The Influence of Medicine on American Literature, 1845–1915*. Stanford, CA: Stanford University Press, 2000.
Davis, Robert Leigh. *Whitman and the Romance of Medicine*. Berkeley: University of California Press, 1997.
De Angleis, Rose. *Between Anthropology and Literature: Interdisciplinary Discourse*. New York: Psychology Press, 2002.
Delafield, Catherine. *Women's Diaries as Narrative in the Nineteenth-Century Novel*. Burlington, VT: Ashgate Publishing, 2009.
Dickens, Charles. *Martin Chuzzlewit*. London: Chapman and Hall, 1844.
Diffley, Kathleen. "Daily Emergency: Civil War Stories of the War Generation." *To Live and Die: Collected Stories of the Civil War, 1861–1876*. Durham: Duke University Press, 2002. 1–24.
———. *Where My Heart Is Turning Ever: Civil War Stores and Constitutional Reform, 1861–1876*. Athens: University of Georgia Press, 1992.
Donawerth, Jane. Introduction. *Rhetorical Theory by Women Before 1900*. Ed. Jane Donawerth. New York: Rowman and Littlefield, 2002. xiii–xlii.
Dorsey, Bruce. *Reforming Men and Women: Gender in the Antebellum City*. Ithaca, NY: Cornell University Press, 2006.
Douglas, Ann. "The War Within a War: Women Nurses in the Union Army." *Civil War History* 18:3 (Sept 1972). 197–212.
Douglass, Frederick. *Frederick Douglass: Selected Speeches and Writings*. Eds. Philip Sheldon Foner and Yuval Taylor. Chicago: Laurence Hill Books, 1999.
———. *The Life and Writings of Frederick Douglass*. Vol. 3. Ed. Philip Sheldon Foner. International Publishers, 1975.
———. *Narrative of the Life of Frederick Douglass, an American Slave*. New York: Penguin Books, 1986.
Dubois, Ellen Carol. *The Elizabeth Cady Stanton–Susan B. Anthony Reader: Correspondence, Writings, Speeches*. Boston: Northeastern University Press, 1992.
Dunbar, Virginia M. Foreword on the Reprint Edition. *Notes on Nursing: What It Is and What It Is Not*. New York: Dover, 1969. xi–xviii.
Dunlap, Julia. "Aunt Patty; or, the Endowment." *Godey's Lady's Book and Magazine*. Oct 1867. 75: 448. 319.
———. *Notes of Hospital Life*. Philadelphia: Lippincott, 1864.
———. "The Four-Footed Orderly." *Boston Recorder*. Aug 5, 1864. xix, 32. 128.
———. "The Four-Footed Orderly." *Stroughton Sentinel*. Aug 27, 1864. 1.

Easley, Alexis. *First-Person Anonymous: Women Writers and Victorian Print Media, 1830–70*. Burlington, VT: Ashgate, 2004.

Eastman, Mary Henderson. *Jenny Wade of Gettysburg*. Philadelphia: Lippincott, 1864.

Eiselein, Gregory. *Literature and Humanitarian Reform in the Civil War Era*. Bloomington: Indiana University Press, 1996.

Eiselein, Gregory, and Anne K. Philips, Eds. *Hospital Sketches*. Westport, CT: Greenwood, 2001. 138–40.

Elbert, Sarah. *A Hunger for Home: Louisa May Alcott's Place in American Culture*. New Brunswick, NJ: Rutgers University Press, 1987.

———. Introduction. *Louisa May Alcott: On Race, Sex, and Slavery*. Boston: Northeastern University Press, 1997. ix–lx.

Elson, Louis Charles. *Modern Music and Musicians for Vocalists: Song Classics*. New York: The University Society, 1918.

Emerson, Ralph Waldo. *Journals and Miscellaneous Notebooks, 1841–1843*. Ed. William Henry Gilman. Cambridge, MA: Belknap Press of Harvard University Press, 1982.

———. *Representative Men: Seven Lectures*. Boston: Phillips, Sampson, and Company, 1856.

Erkkila, Betsy. *Whitman the Political Poet*. New York: Oxford University Press, 1989.

Fabian, Ann. *The Unvarnished Truth: Personal Narratives in Nineteenth-Century America*. Berkeley: University of California Press, 2000.

Fahs, Alice. *The Imagined Civil War: Popular Literature of the North and South, 1861–1865*. Chapel Hill: University of North Carolina Press, 2001.

Faust, Drew Gilpin. *This Republic of Suffering: Death and the American Civil War*. New York: Alfred A. Knopf, 2008.

Fisher, Anna Schall, and Mrs. John Rex. "Anna Morris Holstein, 1824–1900." *Notable Women of Pennsylvania*. Eds. Gertrude Bosler Biddle and Sarah Dickinson Lowre. Philadelphia: University of Pennsylvania Press, 1942. 166–167.

Flannery, Michael A. *Civil War Pharmacy: A History of Drugs, Drug Supply and Provision, and Therapeutics for the Union and Confederacy*. New York: Pharmaceutical Products Press, 2004.

Fleischner, Jennifer. *Mastering Slavery: Memory, Family, and Identity in Women's Slave Narratives*. New York: New York University Press, 1996.

Folsom, Ed. *Walt Whitman's Native Representations*. Cambridge: Cambridge University Press, 1994.

Frankenberg, Ruth. *White Women, Race Matters: The Social Construction of Whiteness*. Minneapolis: University of Minnesota Press, 1993.

———. "The Mirage of an Unmarked Whiteness." *The Making and Unmaking*

of Whiteness. Eds. Rasmussen, Birgit Brander, Eric Kleinenberg, Irene J. Nexica, and Matt Wray. Durham, NC: Duke University Press, 2001. 72–96.
———. "The Critical Study of Whiteness." *Researching Race and Racism*. Eds. Martin Bulmer and John Solomos. New York: Routledge, 2004. 110–18.
Fredrickson, George M. *The Inner Civil War: Northern Intellectuals and the Crisis of the Union*. New York: Harper and Row, 1965.
Freud, Sigmund. "The Uncanny." *The Complete Psychological Writings of Sigmund Freud*. Trans. James Strachey. London: Hogarth Press, 1953. Vol 17. 217–56.
"From the Fifth Infantry." *Detroit Free Press*. Aug 10, 1864. 3.
Furgurson, Ernest B. *Freedom Rising: Washington in the Civil War*. New York: Alfred A. Knopf, 2004.
Garvey, Ellen Gruber. *Writing with Scissors: American Scrapbooks from the Civil War to the Harlem Renaissance*. Oxford: Oxford University Press, 2012.
———. "Imitation Is the Sincerest Form of Appropriation," *Common-Place* 7:3 (Apr 2007) http://www.common-place.org/vol-07/no-03/garvey/
Gates, Henry Louis, Jr. *The Signifying Monkey: A Theory of African-American Literary Criticism*. Oxford: Oxford University Press, 1989.
Genoways, Ted. *Walt Whitman and the Civil War: America's Poet During the Lost Years of 1860–1862*. Berkeley: University of California Press, 2009.
Giesberg, Judith. *Army at Home: Women and the Civil War on the Northern Home Front*. Chapel Hill: University of North Carolina Press, 2009.
———. *Civil War Sisterhood: The U. S. Sanitary Commission and Women's Politics In Transition*. Boston: Northeastern University Press, 2000.
Gillespie, James. *Andersonvilles of the North: The Myths and Realities of Northern Treatment of Civil War Confederate Prisoners*. Denton: University of North Texas Press, 2008.
Gilmore, Michael T. *War on Words: Slavery, Race, and Free Speech in American Literature*. Chicago: University of Chicago Press, 2010.
Ginzberg, Lori D. *Woman and the Work of Benevolence: Morality, Politics, and Class In the Nineteenth-Century United States*. New Haven, CT: Yale University Press, 1990.
Godey's Lady's Book. Oct 1868. 460, 358.
Goldstein, Joshua S. *War and Gender: How Gender Shapes the War System and Vice Versa*. Cambridge: Cambridge University Press, 2003.
Goodheart, Adam. *1861: The Civil War Awakening*. New York: Alfred A. Knopf, 2011.
Griffith, Elisabeth. *In Her Own Right: The Life of Elizabeth Cady Stanton*. New York: Oxford University Press, 1984.
Grimes, Ronald L. *Deeply into the Bone: Reinventing Rites of Passage*. Berkeley: University of California Press, 2002.

Hale, Sarah Josepha Buell. *Woman's Record; Or, Sketches of All Distinguished Women, from the Creation to A.D. 1854*. New York: Harper and Brothers, 1855.
———. *Godey's Lady's Book and Magazine*. Oct 1868. 460. 358.
Hall, Ruth. "A Magic Pen." *Prairie Farmer*. Apr 30, 1864. 13, 18. 314.
Hancock, Cornelia. *South After Gettysburg: Letters of a Civil War Nurse*. Ed. Henrietta Stratton Jaquette. Lincoln: University of Nebraska Press, 1998.
Harris, Sharon M. Introduction. *Women's Early American Historical Narratives*. New York: Penguin, 2003.
———. *Rebecca Harding Davis and American Realism*. Philadelphia: University of Pennsylvania Press, 1991.
Harper's New Monthly Magazine. Review. Nov 1869. 39: 234. 925.
Hawk, Alan. "Behind the Front Lines: Review of *Personal Memoirs of John H. Brinton: Civil War Surgeon, 1861–1865*." (Apr 2, 2011) http://www.amazon.com/Personal-Memoirs-John-Brinton-1861-1865/dp/0809320444
Heglar, Charles J. *Rethinking the Slave Narrative: Slave Marriage and the Narratives of Henry Bibb and William and Ellen Craft*. Westport, CT: Greenwood, 2001.
Hendler, Glenn. *Public Sentiments: Structures of Feeling in Nineteenth-Century American Literature*. Chapel Hill: University of North Carolina Press, 2001.
Hilde, Libra Rose. "Worth a Dozen Men: Women, Nursing, and Medical Care During the American Civil War." Diss., Harvard University, 2003.
Hoeller, Hildegard. *Edith Wharton's Dialogue with Realism and Sentimental Fiction*. Gainesville: University Press of Florida, 2000.
Hoisington, Daniel John, Ed. *My Heart Toward Home: Letters of a Family During the Civil War*. Roseville, MN: Edinborough Press, 2001.
Holstein, Anna Morris. *Three Years in Field Hospitals of the Army of the Potomac*. Philadelphia: Lippincott, 1867.
Holzer, Howard and Mark E. Neely Jr. *Mine Eyes Have Seen the Glory: The Civil War in Art*. New York: Orion Books, 1993.
Hosmer, Margaret and Julia Dunlap. *Under the Holly: Or a Week at Hopeton House*. Philadelphia: Porter and Coates, 1870.
Howe, Mark Antony DeWolfe. *Memoirs of the Life and Services of the Right Reverend Alonzo Potter*. Philadelphia: Lippincott, 1871.
Huspek, Michael. Introduction. *Transgressing Discourses: Communication and the Voice of the Others*. Eds. Michael Huspek and Gary P. Radford. Albany: State University of New York Press, 1997. 1–16.
Jackson Citizen Patriot. June 24, 1870. 5.
———. Jan 21, 1889. 7.
Jacobs, Harriet Ann. *Incidents in the Life of a Slave Girl*. Boston: Published for the Author, 1861.

Johnson, Nan. *Gender and Rhetorical Space in American Life, 1866–1910*. Carbondale: Southern Illinois University Press, 2002.

———. *Nineteenth-Century Rhetoric in North America*. Carbondale: Southern Illinois University Press, 1991.

———. "The Popularization of Nineteenth-Century Rhetoric: Elocution and the Private Learner." *Oratorical Culture in Nineteenth-Century America: Transformations In the Theory and Practice of Rhetoric*. Eds. Gregory Clark and S. Michael Halloran. Carbondale: Southern Illinois University Press, 1993. 139–57.

Jones, Bessie Z. Introduction. *Hospital Sketches*. Cambridge: Belknap Press of Harvard University Press, 1960. vii–xliv.

Judd, Catherine. *Bedside Seductions: Nursing and the Victorian Imagination, 1830–1880*. New York: Palgrave Macmillan, 1998.

Kalisch, Philip A. and Beatrice J. Kalisch. *American Nursing: A History*. New York: Lippincott Williams and Wilkins, 2004.

———. "Reading Women/Women Reading: The Making of Learned Women in Antebellum America." *Reading Acts: U. S. Readers' Interactions with Literature, 1800–1950*. Eds. Barbara Ryan and Amy M. Thomas. Knoxville: University of Tennessee Press, 2002. 53–78.

Kinney, Katherine. "Making Capitol: War, Labor, and Whitman in Washington, D.C." *Breaking Bounds: Whitman and American Cultural Studies*. Eds. Betsy Erkkila and Jay Grossman. New York: Oxford University Press, 1996. 174–89.

Kolodny, Annette. "Inventing a Feminist Discourse: Rhetoric and Resistance in Margaret Fuller's *Woman in the Nineteenth Century*." *Reclaiming Rhetorica: Women in the Rhetorical Tradition*. Ed. Andrea A. Lunsford. Pittsburgh: University of Pittsburgh Press, 1995. 137–66.

Laffrado, Laura. *Uncommon Women: Gender and Representation in Nineteenth-Century U. S. Women's Writing*. Columbus: Ohio State University Press, 2009.

Lanman, Charles. *The Red Book of Michigan: A Civil, Military, and Biographical History*. Detroit: E. B. Smith, 1871.

Lawson, Andrew. *Downwardly Mobile: The Changing Fortunes of American Realism*. New York: Oxford University Press, 2012.

Lee, Julia Sun-Joo. *The American Slave Narrative and the Victorian Novel*. Oxford: Oxford University Press, 2010.

Leonard, Elizabeth D. *Yankee Women: Gender Battles in the Civil War*. New York: Norton, 1994.

Littell's Living Age, June 29, 1867. 830.

Litosseliti, Lia, and Jane Sunderland. "Gender Identity and Discourse Analysis: Theoretical and Empirical Considerations." *Gender Identity and*

Discourse Analysis. Eds. Lia Litosseliti and Jane Sunderland. Philadelphia: John Benjamins, 2002. 1–40.

Locke, E. W. *Three Years in Camp and Hospital*. Boston: George D. Russell and Co., 1870.

Long, Lisa. *Rehabilitating Bodies: Health, History, and the American Civil War*. Philadelphia: University of Pennsylvania Press, 2004.

Loving, Jerome. *Walt Whitman: The Song of Himself*. Berkeley: University of California Press, 1999.

Lunsford, Andrea A. "On Reclaiming Rhetorica." *Reclaiming Rhetorica: Women in the Rhetorical Tradition*. Ed. Andrea A. Lunsford. Pittsburgh: University of Pittsburgh Press, 1995. 3–8

Machor, James L. *Reading Fiction in Antebellum America: Informed Response and Reception Histories, 1820–1865*. Baltimore: Johns Hopkins University Press, 2011.

Maher, Sister Mary Denis. *To Bind Up the Wounds: Catholic Sister Nurses in the U. S. Civil War*. Westport, CT: Greenwood Press, 1989.

Manning, Chandra. *What This Cruel War Was Over: Soldiers, Slavery and the Civil War*. New York: Alfred A. Knopf, 2007.

Massey, Elizabeth. *Bonnet Brigades*. New York: Alfred A. Knopf, 1966.

Masur, Kate. "'A Rare Phenomenon of Philological Vegetation': The Word 'Contraband' and the Meanings of Emancipation in the United States." *Journal of American History* 93:4 (2007). 1050–84.

Mattingly, Carol. *Well-Tempered Women: Nineteenth-Century Temperance Rhetoric*. Carbondale: Southern Illinois University Press, 1998.

McDevitt, Theresa. *Women and the American Civil War: An Annotated Bibliography*. Westport, CT: Greenwood, 2003.

McKay, Charlotte E. *Stories of Hospital and Camp*. Philadelphia, 1876.

McPherson, James M. *Battle Cry of Freedom: The Civil War Era*. Oxford: Oxford University Press, 2003.

Miller, J. Hillis. *Speech Acts in Literature*. Stanford, CA: Stanford University Press, 2001.

Miller, Randall M., Ed. *The Greenwood Encyclopedia of Daily Life in America*. Westport, CT: Greenwood, 2008.

Mitchell, Angelyn. *The Freedom to Remember: Narrative, Slavery, and Gender in Contemporary Black Women's Fiction*. New Brunswick, NJ: Rutgers University Press, 2002.

Moore, Frank. Frank Moore Papers, Duke University Archives. Letter From Elvira J. Powers to Frank Moore, June 11, 1866, encl., "For 'Women of the War.'"

———. *Women of the War: Their Heroism and Self-Sacrifice*. Hartford, CT: S. S. Scranton, 1867.

Morrison, Toni. *Playing in the Dark: Whiteness and the Literary Imagination*. New York: Vintage, 1993.
Mountford, Roxanne. *The Gendered Pulpit: Preaching in American Protestant Spaces*. Carbondale: Southern Illinois University Press, 2003.
Najmi, Samina, and Rajini Srikanth. Introduction. *White Women in Racialized Spaces: Imaginative Transformation and Ethical Action in Literature*. Albany: State University of New York Press, 2002. 1–26.
Nightingale, Florence. *Notes on Nursing: What It Is, and What It Is Not*. Ed. Virginia M. Dunbar. New York: Dover, 1969.
Noble, Mariane. *The Masochistic Pleasures of Sentimental Literature*. Princeton, NJ: Princeton University Press, 2000.
"Notes on the Rebel Invasion of Maryland and Pennsylvania and the Battle of Gettysburg." *The North American Review*. 98 (Jan 1864). 202.
Nünning, Ansgar F. "Reconceptualizing Unreliable Narration: Synthesizing Cognitive and Rhetorical Approaches." *A Companion to Narrative Theory*. Eds. James Phelan and Peter J. Rabinowitz. Oxford: Blackwell, 2005. 89–107.
Oates, Stephen B. *A Woman of Valor: Clara Barton and the Civil War*. New York: Free Press, 1994.
Ober, Josiah. *Political Dissent in Democratic Athens: Intellectual Critics of Popular Rule*. Princeton, NJ: Princeton University Press, 2011.
O'Brien, Tim. *The Things They Carried*. New York: First Mariner Books, 2009.
O'Connell Davidson, Julia. "Metamorphosis? Privatisation and the Restructuring of Management and Labour." *Privatisation and Regulation: A Review of the Issues*. Eds. Peter M. Jackson and Catherine Price. Longman, 1994. 170–97.
Okker, Patricia. *Our Sister Editors: Sarah J. Hale and the Tradition of Nineteenth-Century American Women Editors*. Athens: University of Georgia Press, 1995.
Olney, James. "'I Was Born': Slave Narratives, Their Status as Autobiography and as Literature. *Calalloo* 20 (1984). 46–73.
Palmer, Sarah A. *The Story of Aunt Becky's Army-Life*. New York: John F. Trow, 1867.
Payn, James. "Story-Telling." *Eclectic Magazine of Foreign Literature, Science, and Art*. Ed. Walter Hilliard Bidwel. New York: E. R. Pelton, Leavitt, Throw, 1880. Vol. 32. 312–19.
Penner, Louise. *Victorian Medicine and Social Reform: Florence Nightingale Among the Novelists*. New York: Palgrave Macmillan, 2010.
Pferdehirt, Julia. *More Than Petticoats: Remarkable Michigan Women*. Guilford, CT: Globe Pequot Press, 2007.
Phelps, Elizabeth Stuart. *The Gates Ajar*. London: Sampson Lowe, Son and Marston, 1869.

Phisterer, Frederick. *New York in the War of the Rebellion, 1861–1865*. 3rd ed. Albany: J. B. Lyon, 1912.

Pollak, Vivian R. *The Erotic Whitman*. Berkeley: University of California Press, 2000.

Powers, Elvira J. *Hospital Pencillings; Being a Diary While in Jefferson General Hospital, Jeffersonville, Ind., and Others at Nashville, Tennessee, as Matron and Visitor*. Boston: Edward L. Mitchell, 1866.

Price, Kenneth M. "Journalism Incorporated in *Memoranda During the War*." *Whitman's Memory*. April 16, 2004. http://www.iath.virginia.edu/fdw/volume2/ price/contents.htm

Pritchard, Robert W. *A History of the Episcopal Church*. Harrisburg, PA: Morehouse, 1999.

Quarles, Benjamin. *The Negro in the Civil War*. Boston: Da Capo Press, 1989.

Quarles, Benjamin and Franklin, Vincent P. *The Negro in the Making of America*. New York: Simon and Schuster, 1996.

Quinby, Daniel B., Ed. *Monthly Literary Miscellany*. Detroit: Quinby, Wood, and Russell, 1852. Vols. 6–7.

Reports of Committees of the Senate of the United States, for the Third Session of the Thirty-Seventh Congress. Washington, DC: Government Printing Office, 1863.

Reverby, Susan M. *Ordered to Care: The Dilemma of American Nursing, 1850–1945*. Cambridge: Cambridge University Press, 1987.

Reynolds, David. *Walt Whitman's America: A Cultural Biography*. New York: Alfred A. Knopf, 1995.

Richard, Patricia. *Busy Hands: Images of the Family in Northern Civil War Effort*. New York: Fordham University Press, 2003.

Riss, Arthur. *Race, Slavery, and Liberalism in Nineteenth-Century American Literature*. Cambridge: Cambridge University Press, 2006.

Ritchie, Joy, and Kate Ronald. Introduction. *Available Means: An Anthology of Women's Rhetoric(s)*. Eds. Joy Ritchie and Kate Ronald. Pittsburgh: University of Pittsburgh Press, 2001. xv–xxxi.

Robbins, Sarah. *Managing Literacy, Mothering America: Women's Narratives on Reading and Writing in the Nineteenth Century*. Pittsburgh: University of Pittsburgh Press, 2004.

Roberts, Jessica Forbes. "Reading Slavery and the Civil War: 1861–1865." *Cultural History of Reading*. Ed. Sarah Quay. Westport, CT: Greenwood Press, 2008.

Ropes, Hannah. *Civil War Nurse: The Diary and Letters of Hannah Ropes*. Ed. John R. Brumgardt. Knoxville: University of Tennessee Press, 1980.

Ross, Kristie. "Arranging a Doll's House: Refined Women as Union Nurses." *Divided Houses: Gender and the Civil War*. Eds. Catherine Clinton and Nina Silber. Oxford: Oxford University Press, 1992. 97–113.

Rowlandson, Mary. *A Narrative of the Captivity, Sufferings, and Removes, of Mrs. Mary Rowlandson, Who Was Taken Prisoner by the Indians at the Destruction of Lancaster in 1675*. Clinton: Ballard and Bynner, 1853.

Ryan, Susan M. *The Grammar of Good Intentions: Race and the Antebellum Culture of Benevolence*. Ithaca, NY: Cornell University Press, 2003.

Sanchez-Eppler, Karen. *Touching Liberty: Abolition, Feminism, and the Politics of the Body*. Berkeley: University of California Press, 1993.

Sandusky Register. Apr 6, 1865. Vol. XIV: 256. 3.

Saturday Evening Post. Nov 7, 1863. 3.

Scarry, Elaine. *The Body in Pain: The Making and Unmaking of the World*. New York: Oxford University Press, 1985.

Schultz, Jane E. "Performing Genres: Sarah Edmonds' Nurse and Spy and the Case of the Cross-Dressed Text." *Dressing Up For War: Transformations of Gender and Genre in the Discourse and Literature of War*. Eds. Aránzazu Usandizaga and Andrew Monnickendam. New York: Rodopi, 2001. 73–91.

———, Ed. *This Birth-Place of Souls: The Civil War Nursing Diary of Harriet Eaton*. Oxford: Oxford University Press, 2010.

———. *Women at the Front: Hospital Workers in Civil War America*. Chapel Hill: University of North Carolina Press, 2004.

Searle, John R. *Speech Acts: An Essay in the Philosophy of Language*. Cambridge: Cambridge University Press, 1970.

Seigel, Peggy Brase. "She Went to War: Indiana Women Nurses in the Civil War." *Indiana Magazine of History*. 86:1. (March 1990). 1–27.

Shaver, Lisa. *Beyond the Pulpit: Women's Rhetorical Roles in the Antebellum Religious Press*. Pittsburgh: University of Pittsburgh Press, 2012.

Shiffrin, Steven H. *Dissent, Injustice, and the Meanings of America*. Princeton, NJ: Princeton University Press, 1999.

Showalter, Daniel F. "Disarticulating American Indianness in the National Museum of the American Indian." *Rhetoric, Materiality, and Politics*. Eds. Barbara Biesecker and John Louis Lucaites. New York: Peter Lang, 2009. 253–76.

Showalter, Elaine. Introduction. *Alternative Alcott*. Louisa May Alcott. New Brunswick, NJ: Rutgers University Press, 1988.

Sicherman, Barbara. "Reading and Middle-Class Identity in Victorian America: Cultural Consumption, Conspicuous and Otherwise." *Reading Acts: U. S. Readers' Interactions With Literature, 1800–1950*. Eds. Barbara Ryan

and Amy M. Thomas. Knoxville: University of Tennessee Press, 2002. 137–60.
———. *Well-Read Lives: How Books Inspired a Generation of American Women*. Chapel Hill: University of North Carolina Press, 2010.
Silber, Nina. *Daughters of the Union: Northern Women Fight the Civil War*. Cambridge, MA: Harvard University Press, 2005.
———. "Introduction: Colliding and Collaborating Gender and Civil War Scholarship." *Battle Scars: Gender and Sexuality in the American Civil War*. Eds. Catherine Clinton and Nina Silber. Oxford: Oxford University Press, 2006. 3–18.
———. *The Romance of Reunion*. Chapel Hill: University of North Carolina Press, 1993.
Sizer, Lyde Cullen. *The Political Work of Northern Women Writers and the Civil War, 1850–1872*. Chapel Hill: University of North Carolina Press, 2000.
Smith, Nina Bennett. "The Women Who Went to War: The Union Army Nurse in the Civil War." Diss., Northwestern University, 1981.
Sorisio, Carolyn. *Fleshing Out America: Race, Gender, and the Politics of the Body in American Literature, 1833–1879*. Athens: University of Georgia Press, 2002.
Souder, Emily B. (Mrs. Edmund A.) *Leaves From the Battle-field of Gettysburg: A Series of Letters From a Field Hospital*. Philadelphia: Caxton Press of C. Sherman, 1864.
St. Armand, Barton Levi. *Emily Dickinson and Her Culture: The Soul's Society*. Cambridge: Cambridge University Press, 1986.
Stanton, Elizabeth Cady. *Eighty Years and More (1815–1897): Reminiscences of Elizabeth Cady Stanton*. New York: European Publishing Company, 1898.
Stanton, Elizabeth Cady, Susan B. Anthony, and Matilda Joslyn Gage, Eds. *History of Woman Suffrage*. Rochester: Charles Mann, 1889. Vol I.
Stern, Madeleine B. Introduction. *The Journals of Louisa May Alcott*. Eds. Joel Myserson, Daniel Shealy, and Madeleine B. Stern. Boston: Little, Brown, 1989. 3–39.
———. *Louisa May Alcott: From Blood and Thunder to Hearth and Home*. Boston: Northeastern University Press, 1998.
Stewart, Garrett. *Dear Reader: The Conscripted Audience In Nineteenth-Century British Fiction*. Baltimore: Johns Hopkins University Press, 1996.
Stillé, Charles Janeway. *The United States Sanitary Commission: Being the General Report of Its Work During the War of the Rebellion*. Philadelphia: J. B. Lippincott, 1866.
Stout, Harry S. *Upon the Altar of the Nation: A Moral History of the Civil War*. New York: Penguin, 2007.

Stowe, Harriet Beecher. *Uncle Tom's Cabin; Or Life Among the Lowly*. Vol. II. Boston: John P. Jewett, 1852.

Sweet, Timothy. *Traces of War: Poetry, Photography, and the Crisis of the Union*. Baltimore: Johns Hopkins University Press, 1990.

Syrett, John. "The Confiscation Acts: The North Strikes Back." *An Uncommon Time: The Civil War and the Northern Homefront*. Eds. Paul Alan Cimbala and Randall M. Miller. New York: Fordham University Press, 2002. 280–325.

Taylor, Susie King. *Reminiscences of My Life in Camp: An African American Woman's Civil War Memoir*. Athens: University of Georgia Press, 2006.

Tebbit, Mark. *Philosophy of Law: An Introduction*. New York: Routledge, 2005. *The Independent*. Review. Feb 16, 1865. 17, 846. 2.

Thoreau, Henry David. *The Portable Thoreau*. Ed. Carl Bode. New York: Penguin, 1990.

Time Staff. "The Things They Carry." Time. (Nov 13, 2006). www.time.com/time/magazine/article/0,9171,1558328,00.html.

Tompkins, Jane P. *Sensational Designs: The Cultural Work of American Fiction, 1790–1860*. Oxford: Oxford University Press, 1986.

Tonkovich, Nicole. "Rhetorical Power in the Victorian Parlor: *Godey's Lady's Book* and the Gendering of Nineteenth-Century Rhetoric." *Oratorical Culture in Nineteenth-Century America: Transformations in the Theory and Practice of Rhetoric*. Eds. Gregory Clark and S. Michael Halloran. Carbondale: Southern Illinois University Press, 1993. 158–83.

United States Christian Commission. *United States Christian Commission, for the Army and Navy: Work and Incidents: First Annual Report*. Philadelphia, 1863.

United States Sanitary Commission. *United States Sanitary Commission Bulletin*. Vol. I. New York: The Commission, 1866.

Usandizaga, Aránzazu, and Andrew Monnickendam. Preface. *Dressing Up for War: Transformations of Gender and Genre in the Discourse and Literature of War*. Eds. Aránzazu Usandizaga and Andrew Monnickendam. New York: Rodopi, 2001. ix-xvii.

Venet, Wendy Hamand. *Neither Ballots Nor Bullets: Women Abolitionists and the Civil War*. Charlottesville: University Press of Virginia, 1991.

Wagner, Margaret E., Gary W. Gallagher, and Paul Finkelman, Eds. *The Library of Congress Civil War Desk Reference*. New York: Simon and Schuster, 2009.

Walker, Scott. *Hell's Broke Loose in Georgia: Survival in a Civil War Regiment*. Athens: University of Georgia Press, 2007.

Wardrop, Daneen. "Civil War Nursing Narratives: Whitman's *Memoranda During the War* and Eroticism." *Walt Whitman Quarterly Review* 23 (Summer 2005). 26–47.

———. *Emily Dickinson and the Labor of Clothing*. Lebanon: University Press of New England/University of New Hampshire Press, 2009.

———. *Word, Birth, and Culture in the Poetry of Poe, Whitman, and Dickinson*. Westport, CT: Greenwood Press, 2002.

Washington Reporter. July 26, 1865. LVI: 52. 4.

Wearn, Mary McCartin. *Negotiating Motherhood in Nineteenth-Century American Literature*. New York: Routledge, 2008.

Weinstein, Cindy. *Family, Kinship, and Sympathy in Nineteenth-Century American Literature*. Cambridge: Cambridge University Press, 2004.

Wellman, Judith. *The Road to Seneca Falls: Elizabeth Cady Stanton and the First Woman's Rights Convention*. Chicago: University of Illinois Press, 2004.

Wertheimer, Molly Meijer. "Introduction: Roses in the Snow." *Listening to Their Voices: The Rhetorical Activities of Historical Women*. Ed. Molly Meijer Wertheimer. Columbia: University of South Carolina Press, 1997. 1–15.

Wheelock, Julia S. *The Boys in White: The Experience of a Hospital Agent in and Around Washington*. New York: Lange and Hillman, 1870.

———. Julia Wheelock Collection. 2 Vols.: Journals, photo album, book manuscript, papers. Abraham Lincoln Library and Museum of Lincoln Memorial University.

Wheelwright, Jeff. *The Irritable Heart: The Medical Mystery of the Gulf War*. New York: W. W. Norton, 2001.

Whitman, Walt. *Memoranda During the War*. Ed. Roy P. Basler. Bloomington: Indiana University Press, 1962.

———. *Prose Works 1892*. Ed. Floyd Stovall. New York: New York University Press, 1963. 2 Vols.

Williams, David. *A People's History of the Civil War: Struggles for the Meaning of Freedom*. New York: New Press, 2006.

Williams, Susan S. *Reclaiming Authorship: Literary Women in America, 1850–1900*. Philadelphia: University of Pennsylvania Press, 2006.

Winter, Kari J. *Subjects of Slavery, Agents of Change: Women and Power in Gothic Novels and Slave Narratives, 1790–1865*. Athens: University of Georgia Press, 1992.

Woman's Mission in the Christian Church. Episcopal Church. Diocese of Pennsylvania. Philadelphia: King and Baird, 1864.

Woolsey, Georgeanna. *Three Weeks at Gettysburg*. New York: Anson D. F. Randolph, 1863.

Woolsey, Jane Stuart. *Hospital Days*. New York: Van Nostrand, 1870. (Privately published, 1868.)

Wormeley, Katharine Prescott. *The United States Sanitary Commission: A Sketch of Its Purposes and Its Work*. Boston: Little, Brown, 1863.

Wright, John D. *The Language of the Civil War*. Westport, CT: Greenwood, 2001.
Yellin, Jean Fagan. *Harriet Jacobs: A Life*. New York: Basic Civitas Books, 2004.
Young, Elizabeth. *Disarming the Nation: Women's Writing and the American Civil War*. Chicago: University of Chicago Press, 1999.
Zagarri, Rosemarie. "The Postcolonial Culture of Early American Women's Writing." *The Cambridge Companion to Nineteenth-Century Women's Writing*. Eds. Dale M. Bauer and Philip Gould. Cambridge: Cambridge University Press, 2001. 19–37.
Zion's Herald. Review. Sep 2, 1869. 46, 35. 413.

INDEX